CONTENTS

INTRODUCTION

Welcome to a journey of natural healing and holistic wellness. This book is crafted with care and passion to guide you through the world of natural remedies, offering an extensive collection of treatments that have been cherished for centuries. Our goal is to provide you with accessible, effective, and safe alternatives to conventional medicine, empowering you to take control of your health naturally.

PURPOSE OF THIS BOOK

I wrote this book to bridge the gap between traditional wisdom and modern science, providing a comprehensive resource that highlights the benefits of natural remedies. In a world where synthetic medications dominate, it is essential to remember and utilise the healing power of nature. Our purpose is to bring to light the remarkable effectiveness of natural treatments and how they can be integrated into your daily life to enhance your well-being.

ADVANTAGES OF USING NATURAL REMEDIES

Safety and Fewer Side Effects: Natural remedies, when used correctly, are generally safer and have fewer side effects compared to their synthetic counterparts. Herbs and plants have been used for thousands of years, with many traditional practices proving their efficacy and safety over time.

Holistic Healing: Natural remedies often provide holistic benefits, addressing not just the symptoms but the root cause of health issues. They support overall wellness, balancing the body, mind, and spirit.

Cost-Effective: Many natural remedies are more affordable than prescription medications. They often come from readily available plants and herbs, making them an economical choice for maintaining health.

Sustainable and Eco-Friendly: Using natural remedies supports sustainability and environmental health. By choosing plant-based treatments, we reduce our reliance on chemical pharmaceuticals, which can have detrimental effects on the environment.

DISADVANTAGES OF MAN-MADE ALTERNATIVES

Side Effects and Health Risks: Synthetic medications often come with a long list of side effects. While they can be highly effective for acute conditions, their prolonged use can lead to adverse health effects and dependency.

Chemical Exposure: Man-made drugs often contain synthetic chemicals that can be harsh on the body. These substances can disrupt the natural balance of our body systems, leading to further health complications.

Over-Medication and Resistance: The overuse of antibiotics and other medications has led to the rise of drug-resistant strains of bacteria and other pathogens. This resistance can make infections harder to treat and lead to more severe health crises.

WHY I WROTE THIS BOOK

My passion for natural health and a desire to share this knowledge with others motivated me to write this book. I believe that everyone deserves access to safe, effective, and natural health solutions. This book is a labour of love, designed to provide you with the tools and information you need to make informed decisions about your health.

I hope that this book inspires you to explore the benefits of natural remedies and integrate them into your life. May it serve as a trusted companion on your journey to better health and wellness.

IMMUNE SYSTEM BOOSTERS

Maintaining a strong immune system is crucial for overall health and well-being. Natural remedies such as elderberry and echinacea have long been valued for their ability to enhance immune function and provide relief from various illnesses.

ELDERBERRY

Overview: Elderberry (Sambucus nigra) is celebrated for its immune-boosting properties, thanks to its rich content of essential vitamins and bioactive compounds.

Key Benefits:

- **Vitamin-Rich:** Elderberries are packed with vitamins A, B, and C, all vital for maintaining a robust immune system. Vitamin A supports respiratory health and acts as an antioxidant, while B vitamins are essential for energy production and immune cell function. Vitamin C enhances white blood cell production and combats free radicals.
- **Antiviral Properties:** Elderberry extract has demonstrated the ability to inhibit the replication of viruses, including the influenza virus, making it effective in both preventing and treating flu symptoms.
- **Anti-inflammatory Effects:** The anti-inflammatory properties of elderberry help reduce symptoms such as body aches and fever, commonly associated with colds and flu.

Usage Recommendations:

- **Forms:** Elderberry can be consumed as syrups, gummies, lozenges, and teas.
- **Dosage:** For adults, a preventive dose typically involves 1-2 teaspoons of elderberry syrup daily. During illness, higher doses may be taken every few hours.

ECHINACEA

Overview: Echinacea (Echinacea purpurea, Echinacea angustifolia) is widely recognized for its immune-enhancing, anti-inflammatory, and antioxidant properties.

Key Benefits:

- **Immune System Boost:** Echinacea is commonly used to stimulate the immune system, particularly at the onset of a cold. It increases the production of white blood cells, which are crucial for fighting infections.
- **Anti-inflammatory Properties:** Compounds in echinacea help reduce inflammation, providing relief from symptoms such as sore throat and swelling.
- **Antioxidant Effects:** Echinacea contains antioxidants that protect cells from oxidative stress and free radical damage, promoting overall health.

Usage Recommendations:

- **Forms:** Echinacea is available in capsules, tablets, liquid extracts, and teas.
- **Dosage:** For acute symptoms, adults can take 300 mg of echinacea extract three times daily, or 0.5-1 mL of liquid extract three times daily.

Considerations:

- **Safety:** Both elderberry and echinacea are generally safe when used as directed. However, individuals with autoimmune disorders or allergies to these plants should consult a healthcare provider before use.
- **Interactions:** These supplements may interact with

certain medications, so it's important to consult with a healthcare provider, especially if you are undergoing other treatments.

Conclusion: Elderberry and echinacea are potent natural remedies that can significantly support and enhance the immune system. Elderberry's high vitamin content and antiviral properties make it an excellent choice for flu prevention and treatment. Echinacea's immune-boosting and anti-inflammatory effects are beneficial for reducing the duration and severity of colds. Using these supplements according to recommended dosages can help ensure their effectiveness and safety, contributing to better overall health and resilience against illnesses.

DIGESTIVE HEALTH

Overview: Maintaining digestive health is crucial for overall well-being. Natural remedies like ginger and peppermint have been used for centuries to address various digestive issues. Their effectiveness in easing symptoms such as nausea, pain, inflammation, and gastrointestinal discomfort makes them valuable components of a holistic approach to digestive health.

GINGER

Overview: Ginger (Zingiber officinale) has a long history of use in traditional medicine, spanning over 2,000 years. It is renowned for its effectiveness in treating nausea, pain, and inflammation.

Key Benefits:

- **Nausea Relief:** Ginger is particularly effective in reducing nausea related to pregnancy (morning sickness), surgery, and chemotherapy. It works by stimulating digestive juices and enhancing the digestive process, which helps to alleviate nausea.
- **Anti-inflammatory Properties:** The active compounds in ginger, such as gingerol and shogaol, have strong anti-inflammatory effects. These compounds can help reduce inflammation in the digestive tract, easing discomfort and promoting better digestive health.
- **Pain Relief:** Ginger is also known for its pain-relieving properties, which can be beneficial for various types of gastrointestinal discomfort.

Usage Recommendations:

- **Forms:** Ginger can be consumed in various forms, including fresh, dried, powdered, as a tea, or in supplements.
- **Dosage:** For nausea relief, studies suggest taking 1-1.5 grams of ginger daily. This can be divided into several doses throughout the day for optimal effectiveness.

PEPPERMINT

Overview: Peppermint (Mentha piperita) is another well-regarded natural remedy for digestive health. Its relaxing effects on the gastrointestinal tract make it particularly helpful for conditions such as irritable bowel syndrome (IBS) and other digestive issues.

Key Benefits:

- **IBS Symptom Relief:** Peppermint oil is commonly used to alleviate symptoms of IBS, such as abdominal pain, bloating, and gas. The menthol in peppermint has a relaxing effect on the muscles of the gastrointestinal tract, which helps reduce spasms and discomfort.
- **Digestive Aid:** Peppermint can also help improve the flow of bile, which is essential for the digestion of fats. This can help with overall digestion and reduce symptoms of indigestion.
- **Anti-inflammatory and Antimicrobial Properties:** Peppermint has both anti-inflammatory and antimicrobial properties, which can help maintain a healthy digestive tract and prevent infections.

Usage Recommendations:

- **Forms:** Peppermint can be consumed as a tea, in capsules, or as an essential oil.
- **Dosage:** For IBS relief, enteric-coated peppermint oil capsules are often recommended, as they prevent the oil from being released in the stomach and causing heartburn. The typical dosage is one to two capsules, taken up to three times daily before meals.

Considerations:

- **Safety:** Both ginger and peppermint are generally safe when used as directed. However, individuals with certain conditions, such as gallstones or gastroesophageal reflux disease (GERD), should consult a healthcare provider before use.

- **Interactions:** These remedies may interact with certain medications, so it's important to consult with a healthcare provider, especially if you are taking other treatments.

Conclusion: Ginger and peppermint are highly effective natural remedies for promoting digestive health. Ginger excels in reducing nausea, pain, and inflammation, making it a versatile option for various digestive issues. Peppermint, with its relaxing effects on the gastrointestinal tract, is particularly beneficial for managing IBS and improving overall digestion. Incorporating these natural remedies into your routine, with appropriate dosages and professional guidance, can significantly enhance your digestive health and overall well-being.

SKIN CONDITIONS

Addressing skin conditions effectively often involves using natural remedies known for their therapeutic properties. Tea tree oil and aloe vera are two such remedies, widely recognized for their benefits in treating various skin issues.

TEA TREE OIL

Overview: Tea tree oil (Melaleuca alternifolia) is a powerful essential oil renowned for its antibacterial, antifungal, and anti-inflammatory properties, making it a versatile solution for several skin conditions.

Key Benefits:

- **Acne Treatment:** Due to its strong antibacterial properties, tea tree oil is highly effective against acne-causing bacteria. It helps reduce the severity and number of acne lesions, and its anti-inflammatory effects can also help reduce the swelling and redness associated with acne.
- **Minor Cuts and Wounds:** Tea tree oil can be applied to minor cuts and abrasions to prevent infection and promote faster healing. Its antibacterial properties help keep the wound clean and reduce the risk of bacterial infections.
- **Fungal Infections:** This oil is also effective in treating fungal infections, such as athlete's foot and nail fungus. Its antifungal properties help eradicate the infection and prevent its recurrence.

Usage Recommendations:

- **Application:** Tea tree oil should be diluted with a carrier oil (such as coconut or jojoba oil) before application to avoid skin irritation. A typical dilution is 5-10 drops of tea tree oil per ounce of carrier oil.
- **Frequency:** For acne, apply the diluted mixture to affected areas once or twice daily. For cuts and fungal infections, apply as needed, ensuring the area is kept clean.

ALOE VERA

Overview: Aloe vera (Aloe barbadensis) is widely celebrated for its soothing, moisturising, and healing properties, making it a popular choice for treating various skin irritations and injuries.

Key Benefits:

- **Soothing Burns:** Aloe vera is highly effective in treating burns, including sunburns. Its gel provides a cooling effect, reduces pain and inflammation, and promotes faster healing by stimulating skin regeneration.
- **Healing Cuts and Abrasions:** Aloe vera's antibacterial and anti-inflammatory properties help prevent infection and reduce inflammation in minor cuts and abrasions. It also speeds up the healing process by promoting the production of collagen.
- **Treating Skin Irritations:** Aloe vera is beneficial for a range of skin irritations, including rashes, insect bites, and eczema. Its moisturising properties help soothe dry, irritated skin and provide relief from itching and redness.

Usage Recommendations:

- **Application:** Aloe vera gel can be applied directly from the plant or used in commercially prepared gels. Ensure the product is pure and free from added chemicals or fragrances.
- **Frequency:** For burns and skin irritations, apply aloe vera gel to the affected area several times a day. For cuts and abrasions, use as needed to keep the area moisturised and promote healing.

Considerations:

- **Safety:** Both tea tree oil and aloe vera are generally safe for topical use. However, tea tree oil should always be diluted to prevent skin irritation. Perform a patch test before using these remedies extensively to ensure there are no adverse reactions.

- **Allergies and Sensitivities:** Individuals with sensitive skin or allergies should consult a healthcare provider before using these natural remedies, especially if they have had reactions to other plant-based products.

Conclusion: Tea tree oil and aloe vera are highly effective natural remedies for treating a variety of skin conditions. Tea tree oil excels in managing acne, minor cuts, and fungal infections due to its potent antibacterial and antifungal properties. Aloe vera is renowned for its soothing and healing effects on burns, cuts, and skin irritations. Using these remedies appropriately can enhance skin health and provide relief from various skin issues.

MENTAL HEALTH AND STRESS RELIEF

Mental health and stress relief are critical aspects of overall well-being. Natural remedies such as lavender and chamomile have been traditionally used to help manage anxiety, improve mood, and promote better sleep, in addition to their other therapeutic benefits.

LAVENDER

Overview: Lavender (Lavandula angustifolia) is a popular herb known for its calming and soothing properties. It is widely used in aromatherapy to reduce anxiety, improve mood, and aid sleep, and it also has applications for minor burns and insect bites.

Key Benefits:

- **Anxiety Reduction:** Lavender is commonly used in aromatherapy to help alleviate anxiety and stress. Its calming scent has been shown to lower heart rate and blood pressure, creating a sense of relaxation and tranquillity.
- **Mood Improvement:** Inhalation of lavender essential oil can improve mood and reduce symptoms of depression. Its uplifting properties make it a valuable natural remedy for enhancing emotional well-being.
- **Sleep Aid:** Lavender promotes better sleep quality by creating a relaxing environment. It is especially beneficial for individuals with insomnia or other sleep disorders.
- **Skin Healing:** Beyond its mental health benefits, lavender is also effective for treating minor burns and insect bites. Its anti-inflammatory and antiseptic properties help soothe the skin and promote healing.

Usage Recommendations:

- **Aromatherapy:** Use a few drops of lavender essential oil in a diffuser or inhale directly from the bottle to reduce anxiety and improve mood.
- **Topical Application:** For sleep, add a few drops of lavender

oil to a diffuser or spray on your pillow before bedtime. For skin issues, dilute lavender oil with a carrier oil and apply to the affected area.

CHAMOMILE

Overview: Chamomile (Matricaria chamomilla) is a well-known herb often consumed as tea. It is famous for its calming effects, making it a popular choice for reducing stress and improving sleep quality. Additionally, chamomile has notable anti-inflammatory properties.

Key Benefits:

- **Stress Reduction:** Chamomile tea is widely used to calm the mind and body, helping to reduce stress and anxiety. Its mild sedative effect promotes relaxation without causing drowsiness.
- **Improved Sleep Quality:** Chamomile is a natural sleep aid that can help improve sleep quality and duration. Drinking chamomile tea before bedtime can make it easier to fall asleep and stay asleep.
- **Anti-inflammatory Properties:** Chamomile contains compounds that help reduce inflammation, making it beneficial for soothing digestive issues and skin irritations.

Usage Recommendations:

- **Tea:** To reduce stress and improve sleep, drink a cup of chamomile tea 30 minutes to an hour before bedtime. Steep 1-2 teaspoons of dried chamomile flowers in hot water for 5-10 minutes.
- **Topical Application:** For skin irritations, chamomile can be applied topically as a compress. Soak a cloth in chamomile tea and apply to the affected area.

Considerations:

- **Safety:** Both lavender and chamomile are generally safe for most people. However, individuals with allergies to these plants should exercise caution. It is advisable to perform a patch test when using essential oils topically.
- **Interactions:** These remedies can interact with certain medications. If you are taking other treatments, consult a healthcare provider before use.

Conclusion: Lavender and chamomile are effective natural remedies for managing mental health and stress. Lavender is excellent for reducing anxiety, improving mood, and aiding sleep through aromatherapy. Chamomile, often enjoyed as a tea, is renowned for its stress-relieving and sleep-enhancing properties. Additionally, both remedies offer anti-inflammatory benefits, making them versatile choices for promoting overall well-being. Using these natural remedies as part of your daily routine can significantly contribute to better mental health and stress management.

PAIN RELIEF

Natural remedies such as turmeric and willow bark have been used for centuries to provide effective pain relief. These remedies are known for their anti-inflammatory and analgesic properties, which help in managing pain associated with various conditions.

TURMERIC

Overview: Turmeric (Curcuma longa) is a spice commonly used in cooking and traditional medicine. Its active ingredient, curcumin, is renowned for its potent anti-inflammatory and antioxidant effects, making it highly effective in treating conditions like arthritis and other inflammatory ailments.

Key Benefits:

- **Anti-inflammatory Effects:** Curcumin, the active compound in turmeric, inhibits inflammatory pathways in the body, reducing inflammation and associated pain. This makes it particularly beneficial for conditions such as arthritis, where inflammation is a major symptom.
- **Antioxidant Properties:** Curcumin is also a powerful antioxidant, helping to neutralise free radicals and reduce oxidative stress. This not only aids in pain relief but also promotes overall health by protecting cells from damage.
- **Pain Management:** The combined anti-inflammatory and antioxidant properties of curcumin help in managing chronic pain, making it a natural alternative to conventional pain relievers.

Usage Recommendations:

- **Forms:** Turmeric can be consumed as a spice in food, in supplements, or as a tea. For enhanced absorption, it is often combined with black pepper, which contains piperine, a compound that increases curcumin's bioavailability.
- **Dosage:** For pain relief, a common dosage is 500-2,000 mg of turmeric extract per day, standardised to contain

95% curcuminoids. It is advisable to consult a healthcare provider for the appropriate dosage.

WILLOW BARK

Overview: Willow bark (Salix spp.) has been used for centuries as a natural pain reliever. It contains salicin, a compound that is chemically similar to aspirin and serves as a precursor to it, providing analgesic and anti-inflammatory effects.

Key Benefits:

- **Natural Pain Relief:** Salicin in willow bark is converted into salicylic acid in the body, which helps reduce pain and inflammation. It is particularly effective for conditions such as headaches, muscle pain, and arthritis.
- **Anti-inflammatory Properties:** Willow bark's anti-inflammatory effects make it useful for treating inflammatory conditions like osteoarthritis and rheumatoid arthritis, helping to reduce swelling and improve joint function.
- **Fewer Side Effects:** Compared to synthetic aspirin, willow bark is often considered gentler on the stomach, making it a preferable option for those who experience gastrointestinal issues with conventional pain relievers.

Usage Recommendations:

- **Forms:** Willow bark is available in various forms, including capsules, tablets, teas, and liquid extracts.
- **Dosage:** For pain relief, a typical dose is 120-240 mg of salicin per day, depending on the severity of symptoms and individual tolerance. As always, it is best to consult with a healthcare provider to determine the appropriate dosage.

Considerations:

- **Safety:** Both turmeric and willow bark are generally safe when used as directed. However, individuals with certain medical conditions or those taking specific medications should consult a healthcare provider before use. Turmeric may interact with blood thinners, and willow bark should be avoided by those with aspirin allergies or certain other conditions.

- **Interactions:** These natural remedies can interact with other medications, so it is important to consult a healthcare provider, especially if you are undergoing other treatments.

Conclusion: Turmeric and willow bark are effective natural remedies for pain relief. Turmeric, with its potent anti-inflammatory and antioxidant properties, is particularly beneficial for managing arthritis and other inflammatory conditions. Willow bark, a natural precursor to aspirin, provides reliable pain relief and is especially useful for headaches, muscle pain, and arthritis. Incorporating these natural remedies into your pain management routine, with appropriate dosages and professional guidance, can help alleviate pain and improve quality of life.

RESPIRATORY HEALTH

Natural remedies such as licorice root and thyme have been used for centuries to support respiratory health. These remedies are known for their soothing, antibacterial, and expectorant properties, which help in managing respiratory conditions and alleviating symptoms such as sore throats, coughs, and bronchitis.

LICORICE ROOT

Overview: Licorice root (Glycyrrhiza glabra) is a traditional remedy known for its soothing and healing properties. It is particularly effective in alleviating respiratory discomforts, including sore throats, bronchitis, and coughs.

Key Benefits:

- **Soothes Sore Throats:** Licorice root contains glycyrrhizin, a compound known for its anti-inflammatory and soothing effects. These properties help to coat the throat, reducing irritation and pain associated with sore throats.
- **Eases Symptoms of Bronchitis and Coughs:** The anti-inflammatory properties of licorice root help reduce inflammation in the bronchial tubes, facilitating easier breathing. Its expectorant qualities also assist in loosening and expelling mucus from the respiratory tract, which is beneficial in treating bronchitis and persistent coughs.

Usage Recommendations:

- **Forms:** Licorice root is available in various forms, including teas, lozenges, and capsules. Licorice root tea is particularly effective for soothing sore throats.
- **Dosage:** For respiratory relief, it is recommended to drink licorice root tea up to three times a day. When using supplements or other forms, it is important to follow the dosage instructions on the product label or consult with a healthcare provider.

THYME

Overview: Thyme (Thymus vulgaris) is a well-known culinary herb with significant medicinal properties. Its antibacterial and expectorant characteristics make it highly effective in treating respiratory issues such as coughs and infections.

Key Benefits:

- **Antibacterial Properties:** Thyme contains thymol, a compound with potent antibacterial effects. It helps to combat respiratory infections by eliminating bacteria that can cause illness.
- **Expectorant Effects:** Thyme acts as a natural expectorant, aiding in the loosening and thinning of mucus in the airways. This facilitates the expulsion of mucus from the respiratory tract, providing relief from congestion and improving breathing.

Usage Recommendations:

- **Forms:** Thyme can be used in various forms, including teas, essential oils, and as a culinary herb. Thyme tea and thyme essential oil (used in steam inhalation) are commonly employed for respiratory support.
- **Dosage:** To prepare thyme tea, steep 1-2 teaspoons of dried thyme in hot water for about 10 minutes. It is recommended to drink this tea up to three times daily. For steam inhalation, add a few drops of thyme essential oil to hot water, cover your head with a towel, and inhale the steam for 5-10 minutes.

Considerations:

- **Safety:** Both licorice root and thyme are generally safe when used as directed. However, individuals with certain medical conditions or those taking specific medications should consult a healthcare provider before use. Licorice root can affect blood pressure and hormone levels, and thyme essential oil should be used with caution to avoid allergic reactions.
- **Interactions:** These natural remedies can interact with other medications, so it is important to consult a healthcare provider, especially if you are undergoing other treatments.

Conclusion:

Licorice root and thyme are effective natural remedies for supporting respiratory health. Licorice root is beneficial for soothing sore throats and easing symptoms of bronchitis and coughs due to its anti-inflammatory and expectorant properties. Thyme's antibacterial and expectorant effects make it a valuable remedy for treating coughs and respiratory infections. Incorporating these natural remedies into your wellness routine, with appropriate dosages and professional guidance, can provide significant relief and support for your respiratory system.

CARDIOVASCULAR HEALTH

Maintaining cardiovascular health is crucial for overall well-being and longevity. Natural remedies such as garlic and hawthorn have been used for centuries to support heart health and manage cardiovascular conditions. These remedies are known for their ability to lower blood pressure, improve heart function, and reduce the risk of heart disease.

GARLIC

Overview: Garlic (Allium sativum) is a popular culinary ingredient that has also been used in traditional medicine for its therapeutic properties. It is particularly known for its ability to lower blood pressure and reduce the risk of heart disease due to its anti-inflammatory and antioxidant properties.

Key Benefits:

- **Lowers Blood Pressure:** Garlic helps to relax blood vessels and improve blood flow, which can lead to lower blood pressure. This is largely due to the presence of allicin, a compound released when garlic is crushed or chopped.
- **Reduces Risk of Heart Disease:** The anti-inflammatory and antioxidant properties of garlic help to reduce oxidative stress and inflammation in the body, both of which are risk factors for heart disease. Garlic also helps to lower levels of LDL (bad) cholesterol and increase HDL (good) cholesterol, further contributing to heart health.
- **Improves Circulation:** Garlic enhances circulation by preventing the aggregation of platelets, which can help to prevent blood clots and improve overall cardiovascular function.

Usage Recommendations:

- **Forms:** Garlic can be consumed fresh, as a supplement, or in powdered form. Fresh garlic is particularly potent, but supplements are also available for those who find the taste of fresh garlic too strong.
- **Dosage:** For cardiovascular health, it is recommended to consume one to two cloves of fresh garlic daily. Garlic

supplements should be taken according to the dosage instructions on the product label or as advised by a healthcare provider.

HAWTHORN

Overview: Hawthorn (Crataegus spp.) is a traditional herbal remedy that has been used to improve cardiovascular function. It is particularly effective in treating conditions such as high blood pressure and heart failure.

Key Benefits:

- **Improves Heart Function:** Hawthorn enhances the strength of heart contractions, increases blood flow to the heart muscle, and helps to maintain a regular heartbeat. These effects are beneficial for individuals with heart failure and other cardiovascular conditions.
- **Lowers Blood Pressure:** Hawthorn helps to dilate blood vessels, improving circulation and reducing blood pressure. This makes it useful for managing hypertension.
- **Antioxidant Properties:** Hawthorn is rich in flavonoids and other antioxidants that help to reduce oxidative stress and protect the cardiovascular system from damage.
- **Reduces Symptoms of Heart Failure:** Studies have shown that hawthorn can help to reduce symptoms of heart failure, such as shortness of breath and fatigue, improving quality of life for those with this condition.

Usage Recommendations:

- **Forms:** Hawthorn is available in various forms, including teas, tinctures, and capsules. Hawthorn extract is often standardised to contain specific amounts of active compounds.
- **Dosage:** For cardiovascular support, a typical dosage of hawthorn extract is 160-900 mg per day, divided into two

or three doses. It is important to consult with a healthcare provider to determine the appropriate dosage based on individual health needs.

Considerations:

- **Safety:** Both garlic and hawthorn are generally safe when used as directed. However, individuals with certain medical conditions or those taking specific medications should consult a healthcare provider before use. Garlic can interact with blood thinners and other medications, and hawthorn can interact with heart medications.
- **Interactions:** These natural remedies can interact with other medications, so it is important to consult a healthcare provider, especially if you are undergoing other treatments.

Conclusion:

Garlic and hawthorn are effective natural remedies for supporting cardiovascular health. Garlic, with its potent anti-inflammatory and antioxidant properties, is particularly beneficial for lowering blood pressure and reducing the risk of heart disease. Hawthorn, known for its ability to improve heart function and lower blood pressure, is especially useful for managing conditions like heart failure and hypertension. Incorporating these natural remedies into your heart health routine, with appropriate dosages and professional guidance, can help enhance cardiovascular function and reduce the risk of heart-related conditions.

ENERGY AND VITALITY

Boosting energy and vitality is essential for maintaining a high quality of life, particularly in managing daily tasks and enhancing overall well-being. Natural remedies such as ginseng and maca root have long been used to enhance energy levels, reduce fatigue, and improve both physical and mental performance.

GINSENG

Overview: Ginseng (Panax ginseng) is a traditional herbal remedy widely recognized for its ability to boost energy, reduce fatigue, and enhance mental performance. It has been used in various cultures for centuries, particularly in Asian medicine.

Key Benefits:

- **Increases Energy Levels:** Ginseng is known to stimulate physical and mental activity, particularly in people who are weak and tired. It helps to improve energy metabolism, providing a natural boost in energy.
- **Reduces Fatigue:** By enhancing the body's resistance to physical and mental stress, ginseng helps to reduce feelings of fatigue and improves endurance.
- **Enhances Mental Performance:** Ginseng has been shown to improve cognitive function, including memory, concentration, and mental clarity. This makes it an excellent remedy for enhancing overall mental performance.
- **Supports Immune Function:** Ginseng also has immune-boosting properties, helping to strengthen the body's defence mechanisms and improve overall vitality.

Usage Recommendations:

- **Forms:** Ginseng can be consumed in various forms, including teas, capsules, powders, and extracts.
- **Dosage:** For boosting energy and reducing fatigue, a typical dosage of ginseng extract is 200-400 mg per day. It is advisable to consult with a healthcare provider to determine the appropriate dosage based on individual

needs and health conditions.

MACA ROOT

Overview: Maca root (Lepidium meyenii) is a root vegetable native to the Andes of Peru, traditionally used to enhance energy, stamina, and sexual function. It is often referred to as a superfood due to its rich nutritional profile.

Key Benefits:

- **Enhances Energy and Stamina:** Maca root is known to increase energy levels and improve stamina, making it a popular supplement among athletes and those with active lifestyles.
- **Reduces Fatigue:** By supporting the adrenal glands and balancing hormones, maca root helps to reduce chronic fatigue and boost overall vitality.
- **Improves Sexual Function:** Maca root has been shown to enhance libido and sexual function in both men and women. It supports reproductive health and can improve fertility.
- **Balances Hormones:** Maca helps to regulate hormones, which can be particularly beneficial for women experiencing menopause or menstrual issues.

Usage Recommendations:

- **Forms:** Maca root is available in powder form, capsules, and as a tincture. The powder can be easily added to smoothies, oatmeal, and other foods.
- **Dosage:** For enhancing energy and stamina, a common dose of maca root powder is 1-3 grams per day. As with ginseng, it is best to consult with a healthcare provider to determine the appropriate dosage based on individual

health needs.

Considerations:

- **Safety:** Both ginseng and maca root are generally safe when used as directed. However, individuals with certain medical conditions or those taking specific medications should consult a healthcare provider before use. Ginseng may affect blood sugar levels and blood pressure, while maca root should be used with caution in those with thyroid issues.

- **Interactions:** These natural remedies can interact with other medications and supplements, so it is important to seek medical advice, especially if you are undergoing other treatments.

Conclusion:

Ginseng and maca root are powerful natural remedies for enhancing energy and vitality. Ginseng is particularly effective in boosting energy levels, reducing fatigue, and improving mental performance. Maca root is well-known for increasing stamina, reducing fatigue, and improving sexual function. Incorporating these natural remedies into your daily routine, with appropriate dosages and professional guidance, can help you maintain high energy levels, improve overall vitality, and enhance quality of life.

ANTI-AGING AND LONGEVITY

Promoting anti-aging and longevity is essential for maintaining a high quality of life and preventing chronic diseases. Natural remedies such as resveratrol and ashwagandha are well-regarded for their ability to reduce the effects of ageing and enhance overall vitality. These remedies are known for their powerful antioxidant properties and stress-managing capabilities.

RESVERATROL

Overview: Resveratrol is a potent antioxidant found in grapes, berries, and red wine. It is widely recognized for its anti-aging properties and its ability to reduce the risk of chronic diseases.

Key Benefits:

- **Anti-Aging Properties:** Resveratrol helps to combat the signs of ageing by protecting cells from oxidative stress and damage. It supports healthy skin, reduces wrinkles, and promotes a youthful appearance.

- **Reduces Risk of Chronic Diseases:** The antioxidant properties of resveratrol help to reduce inflammation and prevent the development of chronic diseases such as heart disease, diabetes, and cancer.

- **Improves Cardiovascular Health:** Resveratrol supports heart health by improving endothelial function and reducing the risk of atherosclerosis. It also helps to lower blood pressure and improve cholesterol levels.

- **Enhances Longevity:** Studies suggest that resveratrol may activate certain genes associated with longevity and overall lifespan.

Usage Recommendations:

- **Forms:** Resveratrol can be consumed in its natural form through grapes and berries, or as a dietary supplement. It is also present in red wine, but supplementation is often preferred to avoid alcohol consumption.

- **Dosage:** For anti-aging benefits, a typical dosage of resveratrol supplements ranges from 150-500 mg per day. It is advisable to consult with a healthcare provider to determine the appropriate dosage based on individual health needs.

ASHWAGANDHA

Overview: Ashwagandha (Withania somnifera) is an adaptogenic herb traditionally used in Ayurvedic medicine. It is known for its ability to help the body manage stress and improve overall vitality and longevity.

Key Benefits:

- **Stress Management:** Ashwagandha helps to reduce cortisol levels, the body's primary stress hormone. By managing stress, it promotes mental clarity, reduces anxiety, and improves overall well-being.
- **Enhances Vitality:** Ashwagandha boosts energy levels, enhances physical performance, and supports endurance. It is particularly beneficial for combating fatigue and increasing overall vitality.
- **Supports Immune Function:** The immune-boosting properties of ashwagandha help to protect the body against infections and diseases, contributing to improved health and longevity.
- **Anti-Aging Effects:** Ashwagandha's antioxidant properties help to protect cells from damage and reduce the signs of ageing. It supports healthy skin, reduces the appearance of fine lines and wrinkles, and promotes a youthful complexion.

Usage Recommendations:

- **Forms:** Ashwagandha is available in various forms, including powders, capsules, and tinctures. It can be easily incorporated into the diet or taken as a supplement.
- **Dosage:** For improving overall vitality and managing

stress, a common dosage of ashwagandha extract is 300-600 mg per day. It is best to consult with a healthcare provider to determine the appropriate dosage based on individual health needs.

Considerations:

- **Safety:** Both resveratrol and ashwagandha are generally safe when used as directed. However, individuals with certain medical conditions or those taking specific medications should consult a healthcare provider before use. Resveratrol may interact with blood thinners, and ashwagandha should be used with caution in individuals with autoimmune diseases.
- **Interactions:** These natural remedies can interact with other medications and supplements, so it is important to seek medical advice, especially if you are undergoing other treatments.

Conclusion:

Resveratrol and ashwagandha are powerful natural remedies for promoting anti-aging and longevity. Resveratrol, with its potent antioxidant properties, is particularly effective in reducing the effects of ageing and lowering the risk of chronic diseases. Ashwagandha, known for its adaptogenic properties, helps the body manage stress and enhances overall vitality and longevity. Incorporating these natural remedies into your wellness routine, with appropriate dosages and professional guidance, can help you maintain a youthful appearance, improve vitality, and enhance quality of life.

ALLERGY RELIEF

Managing allergies effectively is essential for maintaining a comfortable and healthy lifestyle. Natural remedies such as stinging nettle and quercetin are well-regarded for their ability to reduce allergic reactions and inflammation, providing relief from common allergy symptoms.

STINGING NETTLE

Overview: Stinging nettle (Urtica dioica) has been traditionally used for its medicinal properties. It acts as a natural antihistamine, making it effective in treating hay fever and other allergic conditions.

Key Benefits:

- **Natural Antihistamine:** Stinging nettle helps to reduce the production of histamines, which are responsible for allergic symptoms such as sneezing, itching, and swelling. By inhibiting histamine production, it alleviates these symptoms.
- **Reduces Inflammation:** The anti-inflammatory properties of stinging nettle help to soothe inflammation in the body, which can be beneficial in managing various allergic reactions.
- **Relieves Hay Fever:** Stinging nettle is particularly effective in treating hay fever, also known as allergic rhinitis. It helps to reduce nasal congestion, runny nose, and itchy eyes.

Usage Recommendations:

- **Forms:** Stinging nettle can be consumed as a tea, in capsules, or as a tincture. Nettle tea is a popular form for allergy relief.
- **Dosage:** For allergy relief, a common dosage is 300-500 mg of stinging nettle extract daily. Drinking nettle tea up to three times a day can also be beneficial. It is advisable to consult a healthcare provider to determine the appropriate dosage based on individual needs.

QUERCETIN

Overview: Quercetin is a natural flavonoid found in many fruits and vegetables, such as apples and onions. It is known for its ability to reduce allergic reactions and inflammation, making it an effective natural remedy for allergy relief.

Key Benefits:

- **Reduces Allergic Reactions:** Quercetin stabilizes mast cells, which are involved in the release of histamines during allergic reactions. By preventing the release of histamines, quercetin helps to reduce the severity of allergic symptoms.
- **Anti-inflammatory Properties:** Quercetin has strong anti-inflammatory effects, which help to reduce inflammation and swelling associated with allergic reactions.
- **Supports Immune Health:** As an antioxidant, quercetin also supports overall immune health, helping the body to respond better to allergens.

Usage Recommendations:

- **Forms:** Quercetin can be consumed through dietary sources such as apples, onions, and berries. It is also available as a supplement in capsules or tablets.
- **Dosage:** For allergy relief, a typical dosage of quercetin supplements is 500-1,000 mg per day, divided into two or three doses. It is best to consult a healthcare provider to determine the appropriate dosage based on individual health needs.

Considerations:

- **Safety:** Both stinging nettle and quercetin are generally safe when used as directed. However, individuals with certain medical conditions or those taking specific medications should consult a healthcare provider before use. Stinging nettle may interact with blood pressure and blood sugar medications, while quercetin may interact with antibiotics and other medications.
- **Interactions:** These natural remedies can interact with other medications and supplements, so it is important to seek medical advice, especially if you are undergoing other treatments.

Conclusion:

Stinging nettle and quercetin are effective natural remedies for managing allergies. Stinging nettle acts as a natural antihistamine, reducing histamine production and alleviating symptoms of hay fever and other allergic reactions. Quercetin, a powerful flavonoid, helps to stabilize mast cells, reduce inflammation, and support overall immune health. Incorporating these natural remedies into your allergy management routine, with appropriate dosages and professional guidance, can provide significant relief and improve quality of life during allergy seasons.

HEADACHES AND MIGRAINES

Effectively managing headaches and migraines is crucial for maintaining daily productivity and overall well-being. Natural remedies such as feverfew and peppermint oil have been traditionally used to alleviate these conditions. These remedies are known for their preventive and therapeutic properties.

FEVERFEW

Overview: Feverfew (Tanacetum parthenium) is a medicinal herb that has been used for centuries to prevent and treat migraines. It contains active compounds that help reduce the frequency and severity of migraine attacks.

Key Benefits:

- **Migraine Prevention:** Feverfew is known for its ability to prevent migraines by inhibiting the release of substances that cause blood vessels to constrict and lead to headaches. Regular use can reduce the frequency and intensity of migraine episodes.
- **Anti-inflammatory Properties:** The anti-inflammatory effects of feverfew help to decrease inflammation in blood vessels, which can contribute to migraine pain.
- **Pain Relief:** Feverfew helps alleviate pain associated with migraines and can be beneficial in reducing symptoms such as nausea and light sensitivity that often accompany migraines.

Usage Recommendations:

- **Forms:** Feverfew is available in various forms, including dried leaves, capsules, tablets, and liquid extracts.
- **Dosage:** For migraine prevention, a typical dosage is 100-300 mg of feverfew extract daily. It is advisable to consult a healthcare provider for the appropriate dosage and duration of use.

PEPPERMINT OIL

Overview: Peppermint oil (Mentha piperita) is widely used for its cooling and soothing properties. When applied topically, it is particularly effective in relieving tension headaches.

Key Benefits:

- **Tension Headache Relief:** The menthol in peppermint oil has a cooling effect that helps to relax and soothe muscles around the head and neck, providing relief from tension headaches.
- **Improves Blood Flow:** Peppermint oil helps to improve blood flow and reduce muscle contractions, which can contribute to headache pain.
- **Quick Acting:** When applied topically, peppermint oil can provide quick relief from headache symptoms.

Usage Recommendations:

- **Forms:** Peppermint oil is primarily used in its essential oil form for topical application.
- **Application:** To relieve tension headaches, dilute a few drops of peppermint oil with a carrier oil (such as coconut or jojoba oil) and apply to the temples, forehead, and back of the neck. Gently massage the oil into the skin. This can be repeated several times a day as needed.

Considerations:

- **Safety:** Both feverfew and peppermint oil are generally safe when used as directed. However, individuals with certain medical conditions or those taking specific medications should consult a healthcare provider before use. Pregnant women should avoid feverfew as it can stimulate uterine contractions.

- **Allergic Reactions:** Some people may experience allergic reactions to feverfew or peppermint oil. A patch test is recommended for peppermint oil to ensure there is no skin irritation or sensitivity.

Conclusion:

Feverfew and peppermint oil are effective natural remedies for managing headaches and migraines. Feverfew is particularly beneficial for preventing migraines and reducing their severity, thanks to its anti-inflammatory and pain-relieving properties. Peppermint oil, with its cooling and soothing effects, provides quick relief from tension headaches when applied topically. Incorporating these natural remedies into your headache and migraine management routine, with appropriate dosages and professional guidance, can help alleviate pain and improve your quality of life.

JOINT AND MUSCLE PAIN

Effectively managing joint and muscle pain is essential for maintaining mobility and overall quality of life. Natural remedies such as arnica and capsaicin have been traditionally used to alleviate pain and reduce inflammation. These remedies are known for their topical applications and ability to provide targeted relief.

ARNICA

Overview: Arnica (Arnica montana) is a well-known herb used in traditional medicine to treat a variety of ailments. It is particularly effective when used topically to reduce inflammation and pain associated with bruises, sprains, and muscle aches.

Key Benefits:

- **Reduces Inflammation:** Arnica contains compounds like sesquiterpene lactones, which help to reduce inflammation and swelling in the affected area.
- **Pain Relief:** The analgesic properties of arnica make it effective in relieving pain from injuries such as bruises, sprains, and muscle aches.
- **Improves Healing:** Arnica promotes the healing process by increasing blood flow to the affected area, which helps to deliver essential nutrients and remove waste products.

Usage Recommendations:

- **Forms:** Arnica is available in various topical forms, including gels, creams, ointments, and sprays. It is also available as a homeopathic remedy.
- **Application:** For joint and muscle pain, apply arnica gel or cream to the affected area two to three times daily. It is important to use arnica only on unbroken skin and to avoid contact with mucous membranes and eyes.

CAPSAICIN

Overview: Capsaicin is the active component found in chili peppers (Capsicum spp.) and is used in topical creams and ointments to relieve pain by reducing substance P, a neurotransmitter involved in the sensation of pain.

Key Benefits:

- **Pain Reduction:** Capsaicin helps to relieve pain by depleting substance P, which is responsible for transmitting pain signals to the brain. This reduces the sensation of pain in the affected area.
- **Anti-inflammatory Properties:** Capsaicin also has anti-inflammatory effects, which help to reduce swelling and discomfort in joints and muscles.
- **Effective for Chronic Pain:** Capsaicin is particularly beneficial for chronic pain conditions such as arthritis, neuropathy, and post-herpetic neuralgia.

Usage Recommendations:

- **Forms:** Capsaicin is available in various topical forms, including creams, gels, and patches.
- **Application:** Apply capsaicin cream to the affected area up to four times daily. It is important to wash hands thoroughly after application and avoid contact with eyes, mouth, and other sensitive areas. Initial use may cause a burning sensation, which usually diminishes with continued use.

Considerations:

- **Safety:** Both arnica and capsaicin are generally safe

when used as directed. However, individuals with certain medical conditions or those taking specific medications should consult a healthcare provider before use. Arnica should not be applied to broken skin, and capsaicin should be used with caution to avoid irritation.

- **Allergic Reactions:** Some people may experience allergic reactions or skin sensitivity to arnica or capsaicin. A patch test is recommended to ensure there is no adverse reaction before extensive use.

Conclusion:

Arnica and capsaicin are effective natural remedies for managing joint and muscle pain. Arnica is particularly beneficial for reducing inflammation and pain associated with bruises, sprains, and muscle aches. Capsaicin provides relief by reducing substance P, which helps to lower the sensation of pain and reduce inflammation. Incorporating these natural remedies into your pain management routine, with appropriate applications and professional guidance, can help alleviate pain and improve your quality of life.

COLD AND FLU

Natural remedies such as ginseng and elderflower have been used to effectively manage cold and flu symptoms. These remedies are known for their immune-boosting and symptom-relieving properties, which help in reducing the severity and duration of illness.

GINSENG

Overview: Ginseng (Panax ginseng) is a renowned herbal remedy known for its immune-boosting properties. It is particularly effective in helping the body fend off colds and flu by enhancing immune system function.

Key Benefits:

- **Boosts Immune System:** Ginseng stimulates the production of immune cells, including T-cells, natural killer cells, and macrophages. This helps the body to effectively combat infections.
- **Reduces Cold and Flu Duration:** Regular use of ginseng can help shorten the duration of colds and flu by enhancing the body's ability to fight off the virus.
- **Improves Overall Vitality:** Ginseng not only boosts immune function but also increases energy levels and reduces fatigue, helping you recover more quickly from illness.

Usage Recommendations:

- **Forms:** Ginseng is available in various forms, including capsules, tablets, teas, and extracts.
- **Dosage:** For boosting the immune system, a typical dosage of ginseng extract is 200-400 mg per day. It is advisable to consult a healthcare provider for the appropriate dosage and duration of use.

ELDERFLOWER

Overview: Elderflower (Sambucus nigra) is a traditional remedy known for its ability to reduce the severity and duration of cold symptoms. It is particularly effective due to its anti-inflammatory and antiviral properties.

Key Benefits:

- **Reduces Severity of Symptoms:** Elderflower helps to alleviate common cold symptoms such as nasal congestion, sore throat, and fever. Its anti-inflammatory properties help reduce swelling and irritation in the respiratory tract.
- **Shortens Illness Duration:** Regular use of elderflower can help to shorten the duration of colds by enhancing the body's immune response to viral infections.
- **Antiviral Properties:** Elderflower contains bioactive compounds that have antiviral effects, helping to prevent the spread of viruses within the body.

Usage Recommendations:

- **Forms:** Elderflower is available in various forms, including teas, syrups, tinctures, and capsules.
- **Dosage:** To reduce the severity and duration of cold symptoms, it is recommended to drink elderflower tea up to three times daily or follow the dosage instructions on elderflower supplements or syrups. Consulting a healthcare provider for specific dosage recommendations is advisable.

Considerations:

- **Safety:** Both ginseng and elderflower are generally safe when used as directed. However, individuals with certain medical conditions or those taking specific medications should consult a healthcare provider before use. Ginseng may affect blood sugar levels and blood pressure, while elderflower should be used with caution in individuals with autoimmune conditions.
- **Interactions:** These natural remedies can interact with other medications and supplements, so it is important to seek medical advice, especially if you are undergoing other treatments.

Conclusion:

Ginseng and elderflower are effective natural remedies for managing colds and flu. Ginseng boosts the immune system, helping to fend off infections and reduce the duration of illness. Elderflower is particularly effective in reducing the severity of symptoms and shortening the duration of colds due to its anti-inflammatory and antiviral properties. Incorporating these natural remedies into your cold and flu management routine, with appropriate dosages and professional guidance, can help alleviate symptoms and improve your recovery time.

DIGESTION AND STOMACH ISSUES

Natural remedies such as slippery elm and marshmallow root have been traditionally used to support digestive health and alleviate stomach issues. These remedies are known for their soothing properties, which help in managing conditions such as GERD and ulcers by coating and protecting the digestive tract.

SLIPPERY ELM

Overview: Slippery elm (Ulmus rubra) is a tree native to North America whose inner bark is used for its medicinal properties. It is particularly effective in soothing the digestive tract and treating conditions like GERD (gastroesophageal reflux disease) and ulcers.

Key Benefits:

- **Soothes the Digestive Tract:** Slippery elm contains mucilage, a gel-like substance that coats and soothes the lining of the digestive tract, reducing irritation and inflammation.
- **Treats GERD and Ulcers:** By coating the esophagus and stomach lining, slippery elm helps to protect these areas from acid, reducing symptoms of GERD and promoting the healing of ulcers.
- **Promotes Healing:** Slippery elm's soothing effect can help to promote the healing of irritated or inflamed tissues in the digestive tract.

Usage Recommendations:

- **Forms:** Slippery elm is available in various forms, including powder, capsules, lozenges, and extracts.
- **Dosage:** For digestive relief, a common recommendation is to mix 1-2 tablespoons of slippery elm powder in water and drink it up to three times daily. It is advisable to consult a healthcare provider for the appropriate dosage and form.

MARSHMALLOW ROOT

Overview: Marshmallow root (Althaea officinalis) is a perennial herb known for its high mucilage content, which provides a protective and soothing effect on the digestive tract.

Key Benefits:

- **Coats and Soothes the Digestive Tract:** The mucilage in marshmallow root forms a protective layer on the lining of the digestive tract, which helps to soothe irritation and reduce inflammation.
- **Treats Stomach Issues:** Marshmallow root is effective in managing conditions such as gastritis, ulcers, and inflammatory bowel diseases by reducing irritation and promoting healing.
- **Relieves GERD Symptoms:** By coating the esophagus, marshmallow root helps to reduce the burning sensation and discomfort associated with GERD.

Usage Recommendations:

- **Forms:** Marshmallow root is available in various forms, including teas, capsules, tinctures, and extracts.
- **Dosage:** For digestive issues, it is recommended to drink marshmallow root tea up to three times daily or take 2-5 ml of tincture three times daily. Consulting a healthcare provider for specific dosage recommendations is advisable.

Considerations:

- **Safety:** Both slippery elm and marshmallow root are generally safe when used as directed. However, individuals with certain medical conditions or those taking specific medications should consult a healthcare provider before use. Pregnant and breastfeeding women should also seek medical advice before using these remedies.
- **Interactions:** These natural remedies can interact with other medications by coating the digestive tract and potentially affecting absorption. It is important to seek medical advice, especially if you are taking other treatments.

Conclusion:

Slippery elm and marshmallow root are effective natural remedies for supporting digestive health and managing stomach issues. Slippery elm soothes the digestive tract and helps treat conditions like GERD and ulcers by coating and protecting the lining. Marshmallow root, with its high mucilage content, provides a similar protective and soothing effect, helping to manage gastritis, ulcers, and GERD symptoms. Incorporating these natural remedies into your digestive health routine, with appropriate dosages and professional guidance, can help alleviate symptoms and promote overall digestive wellness.

SKIN CARE

Taking care of your skin is essential for overall health and well-being. Natural remedies such as calendula and neem have been traditionally used to treat various skin conditions. These remedies are known for their anti-inflammatory, healing, and antibacterial properties, which help in managing wounds, skin irritations, acne, and other skin issues.

CALENDULA

Overview: Calendula (Calendula officinalis), also known as marigold, is a plant with bright orange and yellow flowers. It is widely used in creams and ointments for its powerful anti-inflammatory and healing properties, making it particularly effective for treating wounds and skin irritations.

Key Benefits:

- **Anti-inflammatory Properties:** Calendula helps to reduce inflammation in the skin, which can alleviate redness, swelling, and discomfort associated with various skin conditions.

- **Healing and Regenerative Effects:** Calendula promotes the healing of wounds, cuts, and abrasions by stimulating collagen production and increasing blood flow to the affected area.

- **Soothes Skin Irritations:** Calendula is effective in treating skin irritations such as eczema, dermatitis, and rashes, providing relief from itching and irritation.

Usage Recommendations:

- **Forms:** Calendula is available in various forms, including creams, ointments, salves, and oils.

- **Application:** For skin irritations and wound healing, apply calendula cream or ointment to the affected area two to three times daily. It is important to use products that contain a high concentration of calendula extract for maximum effectiveness.

NEEM

Overview: Neem (Azadirachta indica) is a tree native to India, known for its potent antibacterial properties. It is commonly used in skin care to treat acne and other skin conditions due to its ability to combat bacteria and reduce inflammation.

Key Benefits:

- **Antibacterial Properties:** Neem is highly effective in killing bacteria that can cause acne and other skin infections. It helps to keep the skin clear and prevent breakouts.
- **Anti-inflammatory Effects:** Neem reduces inflammation and swelling in the skin, which can help to soothe irritated and inflamed skin conditions such as acne, eczema, and psoriasis.
- **Supports Skin Health:** Neem contains fatty acids and vitamin E, which nourish and moisturize the skin, promoting overall skin health and reducing the appearance of scars and blemishes.

Usage Recommendations:

- **Forms:** Neem is available in various forms, including oils, creams, soaps, and powders.
- **Application:** For acne and skin conditions, apply neem oil or cream to the affected areas once or twice daily. Neem soap can be used as a regular cleanser to maintain clear and healthy skin.

Considerations:

- **Safety:** Both calendula and neem are generally safe

when used as directed. However, individuals with certain medical conditions or those taking specific medications should consult a healthcare provider before use. Calendula should be used with caution by individuals who are allergic to plants in the Asteraceae family.

- **Allergic Reactions:** Some people may experience allergic reactions to calendula or neem. It is advisable to perform a patch test before using these remedies extensively.

Conclusion:

Calendula and neem are effective natural remedies for skin care. Calendula, with its anti-inflammatory and healing properties, is particularly beneficial for treating wounds and skin irritations. Neem, known for its antibacterial properties, is highly effective in treating acne and other skin conditions. Incorporating these natural remedies into your skin care routine, with appropriate applications and professional guidance, can help maintain healthy, clear, and irritation-free skin.

ANXIETY AND DEPRESSION

Managing anxiety and depression is crucial for mental health and overall well-being. Natural remedies such as St. John's Wort and Valerian Root have been traditionally used to alleviate symptoms of anxiety and depression. These remedies are known for their mood-enhancing and calming properties, which help improve mental health and sleep quality.

St. John's Wort

Overview: St. John's Wort (Hypericum perforatum) is a flowering plant widely used in herbal medicine to treat mild to moderate depression. It is recognized for its ability to enhance mood and alleviate symptoms of depression.

Key Benefits:

- **Treats Mild to Moderate Depression:** St. John's Wort is effective in reducing symptoms of mild to moderate depression. It works by increasing the levels of neurotransmitters such as serotonin, dopamine, and norepinephrine in the brain, which help improve mood and emotional balance.
- **Mood Enhancement:** By stabilizing mood and reducing feelings of sadness and hopelessness, St. John's Wort can significantly improve the quality of life for individuals with depression.
- **Reduces Anxiety:** St. John's Wort also helps to alleviate anxiety symptoms, providing a calming effect and

reducing stress levels.

Usage Recommendations:

- **Forms:** St. John's Wort is available in various forms, including capsules, tablets, teas, and liquid extracts.
- **Dosage:** For treating depression, a typical dosage of St. John's Wort extract is 300 mg taken three times daily. It is important to consult a healthcare provider for the appropriate dosage and duration of use.

VALERIAN ROOT

Overview: Valerian Root (Valeriana officinalis) is a perennial herb known for its sedative and calming properties. It is commonly used to reduce anxiety and improve sleep quality, making it beneficial for those experiencing anxiety-related sleep disturbances.

Key Benefits:

- **Reduces Anxiety:** Valerian Root helps to reduce anxiety by increasing the levels of gamma-aminobutyric acid (GABA) in the brain, a neurotransmitter that promotes relaxation and reduces nervous tension.
- **Improves Sleep Quality:** Valerian Root is highly effective in improving sleep quality and duration. It helps individuals fall asleep faster and enjoy a deeper, more restorative sleep.
- **Calming Effect:** The calming properties of Valerian Root help to reduce stress and promote a sense of tranquility, making it beneficial for individuals with anxiety disorders.

Usage Recommendations:

- **Forms:** Valerian Root is available in various forms, including capsules, tablets, teas, and tinctures.
- **Dosage:** For reducing anxiety and improving sleep, a common dosage is 400-600 mg of Valerian Root extract taken 30 minutes to two hours before bedtime. It is advisable to consult a healthcare provider for specific dosage recommendations.

Considerations:

- **Safety:** Both St. John's Wort and Valerian Root are generally safe when used as directed. However, individuals with certain medical conditions or those taking specific medications should consult a healthcare provider before use. St. John's Wort can interact with various medications, including antidepressants, birth control pills, and blood thinners.
- **Side Effects:** Some people may experience side effects such as digestive upset, headache, or dizziness. It is important to monitor your body's response and consult a healthcare provider if any adverse effects occur.

Conclusion:

St. John's Wort and Valerian Root are effective natural remedies for managing anxiety and depression. St. John's Wort is particularly beneficial for treating mild to moderate depression and enhancing mood, while Valerian Root helps reduce anxiety and improve sleep quality. Incorporating these natural remedies into your mental health routine, with appropriate dosages and professional guidance, can help alleviate symptoms and improve overall well-being.

MENSTRUAL AND REPRODUCTIVE HEALTH

Natural remedies such as chasteberry and dong quai have been traditionally used to support menstrual and reproductive health. These remedies are known for their ability to balance hormones, regulate menstrual cycles, and alleviate symptoms associated with PMS, menopause, and menstrual cramps.

CHASTEBERRY

Overview: Chasteberry (Vitex agnus-castus) is a fruit-bearing shrub that has been used for centuries to treat a variety of female reproductive health issues. It is particularly effective in balancing hormones and alleviating symptoms of PMS and menopause.

Key Benefits:

- **Balances Hormones:** Chasteberry helps to regulate the production of hormones, particularly prolactin, which can influence menstrual cycle regularity and alleviate symptoms of PMS.
- **Alleviates PMS Symptoms:** Chasteberry is effective in reducing symptoms of premenstrual syndrome (PMS) such as breast tenderness, mood swings, and irritability.
- **Eases Menopause Symptoms:** Chasteberry can help to balance hormone levels during menopause, reducing symptoms such as hot flashes, night sweats, and mood changes.

Usage Recommendations:

- **Forms:** Chasteberry is available in various forms, including capsules, tablets, tinctures, and extracts.
- **Dosage:** For balancing hormones and alleviating PMS and menopause symptoms, a typical dosage is 20-40 mg of chasteberry extract daily. It is advisable to consult a healthcare provider for the appropriate dosage and duration of use.

DONG QUAI

Overview: Dong Quai (Angelica sinensis) is a traditional Chinese herb known as the "female ginseng." It has been used for centuries to regulate the menstrual cycle, relieve menstrual cramps, and support overall reproductive health.

Key Benefits:

- **Regulates Menstrual Cycle:** Dong Quai helps to regulate the menstrual cycle by promoting blood circulation and balancing hormone levels.
- **Relieves Menstrual Cramps:** The antispasmodic properties of Dong Quai help to alleviate menstrual cramps and reduce discomfort associated with menstruation.
- **Supports Reproductive Health:** Dong Quai is used to improve overall reproductive health, including enhancing fertility and alleviating symptoms of menopause.

Usage Recommendations:

- **Forms:** Dong Quai is available in various forms, including capsules, tablets, teas, and tinctures.
- **Dosage:** For regulating the menstrual cycle and relieving menstrual cramps, a common dosage is 500-1,000 mg of Dong Quai root extract taken daily. It is best to consult a healthcare provider for specific dosage recommendations.

Considerations:

- **Safety:** Both chasteberry and Dong Quai are generally safe when used as directed. However, individuals with certain medical conditions or those taking specific medications should consult a healthcare provider before use. Chasteberry may interact with hormonal therapies, and Dong Quai should be used with caution by individuals with bleeding disorders or those taking blood-thinning medications.

- **Side Effects:** Some people may experience side effects such as digestive upset, headache, or skin reactions. It is important to monitor your body's response and consult a healthcare provider if any adverse effects occur.

Conclusion:

Chasteberry and Dong Quai are effective natural remedies for supporting menstrual and reproductive health. Chasteberry helps to balance hormones and alleviate symptoms of PMS and menopause, while Dong Quai is beneficial for regulating the menstrual cycle and relieving menstrual cramps. Incorporating these natural remedies into your health routine, with appropriate dosages and professional guidance, can help maintain hormonal balance and improve overall reproductive health.

HEART HEALTH

Maintaining heart health is crucial for overall well-being and longevity. Natural remedies such as red yeast rice and cayenne pepper have been traditionally used to support cardiovascular health. These remedies are known for their ability to lower cholesterol levels, improve circulation, and enhance overall heart function.

RED YEAST RICE

Overview: Red yeast rice is a traditional Chinese remedy made by fermenting rice with a specific type of yeast (Monascus purpureus). It contains compounds, including monacolin K, which is chemically identical to the active ingredient in certain cholesterol-lowering medications.

Key Benefits:

- **Lowers Cholesterol:** Red yeast rice is particularly effective in reducing levels of LDL (bad) cholesterol and total cholesterol in the blood. Monacolin K works by inhibiting the enzyme responsible for cholesterol production in the liver.

- **Supports Heart Health:** By lowering cholesterol levels, red yeast rice helps to reduce the risk of heart disease and maintain overall cardiovascular health.

- **Anti-inflammatory Properties:** Red yeast rice also has anti-inflammatory effects that can help to reduce inflammation in the blood vessels, further supporting heart health.

Usage Recommendations:

- **Forms:** Red yeast rice is available in various forms, including capsules and tablets.

- **Dosage:** For lowering cholesterol, a common dosage is 1,200-2,400 mg of red yeast rice extract per day, taken in divided doses. It is advisable to consult a healthcare provider for the appropriate dosage and duration of use.

CAYENNE PEPPER

Overview: Cayenne pepper (Capsicum annuum) is a type of chili pepper known for its spicy flavor and medicinal properties. It contains capsaicin, which is responsible for its health benefits, including improving circulation and reducing cholesterol levels.

Key Benefits:

- **Improves Circulation:** Cayenne pepper helps to improve blood flow and circulation by dilating blood vessels and reducing blood pressure. This can help to prevent blood clots and reduce the risk of heart disease.
- **Reduces Cholesterol Levels:** The capsaicin in cayenne pepper helps to lower LDL (bad) cholesterol and triglycerides, promoting better heart health.
- **Anti-inflammatory Effects:** Cayenne pepper has anti-inflammatory properties that help to reduce inflammation in the blood vessels, supporting overall cardiovascular health.

Usage Recommendations:

- **Forms:** Cayenne pepper is available in various forms, including fresh, dried, capsules, and tinctures.
- **Dosage:** For heart health, a common recommendation is to consume 30-120 mg of cayenne pepper in capsule form daily, or to add fresh or dried cayenne pepper to food. It is best to consult a healthcare provider for specific dosage recommendations.

Considerations:

- **Safety:** Both red yeast rice and cayenne pepper are

generally safe when used as directed. However, individuals with certain medical conditions or those taking specific medications should consult a healthcare provider before use. Red yeast rice can interact with cholesterol-lowering medications, and cayenne pepper may cause stomach irritation or interact with blood-thinning medications.

- **Side Effects:** Some people may experience side effects such as digestive upset or skin irritation. It is important to monitor your body's response and consult a healthcare provider if any adverse effects occur.

Conclusion:

Red yeast rice and cayenne pepper are effective natural remedies for supporting heart health. Red yeast rice helps to lower cholesterol levels and reduce the risk of heart disease, while cayenne pepper improves circulation and reduces cholesterol levels. Incorporating these natural remedies into your heart health routine, with appropriate dosages and professional guidance, can help maintain cardiovascular health and enhance overall well-being.

DIABETES MANAGEMENT

Managing diabetes effectively is essential for maintaining overall health and preventing complications. Natural remedies such as bitter melon and fenugreek have been traditionally used to help control blood sugar levels. These remedies are known for their ability to enhance insulin sensitivity and reduce blood sugar levels, supporting overall diabetes management.

BITTER MELON

Overview: Bitter melon (Momordica charantia) is a tropical fruit widely used in traditional medicine for its ability to lower blood sugar levels. It contains compounds that mimic insulin and help to regulate glucose metabolism.

Key Benefits:

- **Lowers Blood Sugar Levels:** Bitter melon contains active compounds such as charantin, vicine, and polypeptide-p, which help to reduce blood sugar levels. These compounds work by increasing glucose uptake and improving insulin sensitivity.
- **Improves Glucose Metabolism:** Bitter melon helps to enhance the body's ability to metabolize glucose, reducing the amount of sugar in the bloodstream.
- **Antioxidant Properties:** Bitter melon also has antioxidant properties that help to protect cells from damage caused by high blood sugar levels, supporting overall health.

Usage Recommendations:

- **Forms:** Bitter melon is available in various forms, including fresh, juice, capsules, and extracts.
- **Dosage:** For blood sugar control, a common recommendation is to take 50-100 ml of bitter melon juice daily or 500-1,000 mg of bitter melon extract in capsule form. It is advisable to consult a healthcare provider for the appropriate dosage and form.

FENUGREEK

Overview: Fenugreek (Trigonella foenum-graecum) is a herb commonly used in cooking and traditional medicine. It is known for its ability to enhance insulin sensitivity and reduce blood sugar levels, making it beneficial for managing diabetes.

Key Benefits:

- **Enhances Insulin Sensitivity:** Fenugreek seeds contain soluble fiber and compounds such as 4-hydroxyisoleucine that help to improve insulin sensitivity, allowing the body to use insulin more effectively.
- **Reduces Blood Sugar Levels:** Fenugreek helps to lower blood sugar levels by slowing the absorption of carbohydrates and sugars in the digestive tract, leading to more stable blood glucose levels.
- **Supports Digestive Health:** The fiber content in fenugreek also supports digestive health, which can be beneficial for overall metabolic function and weight management.

Usage Recommendations:

- **Forms:** Fenugreek is available in various forms, including seeds, powder, capsules, and extracts.
- **Dosage:** For diabetes management, a common dosage is 2-5 grams of fenugreek seeds daily or 500-1,000 mg of fenugreek extract in capsule form. It is best to consult a healthcare provider for specific dosage recommendations.

Considerations:

- **Safety:** Both bitter melon and fenugreek are generally safe when used as directed. However, individuals with certain medical conditions or those taking specific medications should consult a healthcare provider before use. Bitter melon should be used with caution by individuals with hypoglycemia, and fenugreek may cause gastrointestinal discomfort in some people.

- **Interactions:** These natural remedies can interact with other medications, particularly those used to lower blood sugar levels. It is important to seek medical advice to avoid potential interactions and ensure safe use.

Conclusion:

Bitter melon and fenugreek are effective natural remedies for managing diabetes. Bitter melon helps to lower blood sugar levels and improve glucose metabolism, while fenugreek enhances insulin sensitivity and reduces blood sugar levels. Incorporating these natural remedies into your diabetes management routine, with appropriate dosages and professional guidance, can help maintain stable blood glucose levels and support overall health.

EYE HEALTH

Maintaining good eye health is crucial for overall well-being and quality of life. Natural remedies such as bilberry and eyebright have been traditionally used to support eye health and treat various eye disorders. These remedies are known for their ability to improve vision and alleviate eye irritations.

BILBERRY

Overview: Bilberry (Vaccinium myrtillus) is a fruit closely related to the blueberry and is renowned for its beneficial effects on eye health. It contains high levels of antioxidants, particularly anthocyanins, which help improve vision and treat eye disorders.

Key Benefits:

- **Improves Vision:** Bilberry enhances night vision and overall visual acuity by improving blood circulation to the eyes and strengthening the capillaries.
- **Treats Eye Disorders:** Bilberry is used to manage and treat eye conditions such as glaucoma and cataracts. Its antioxidant properties help to protect the eyes from oxidative stress and damage.
- **Reduces Eye Fatigue:** Bilberry can help reduce eye strain and fatigue, especially for individuals who spend long hours in front of screens or performing tasks that require intense visual focus.

Usage Recommendations:

- **Forms:** Bilberry is available in various forms, including fresh berries, juice, capsules, and extracts.
- **Dosage:** For eye health, a common dosage is 80-160 mg of bilberry extract standardized to contain 25% anthocyanins, taken once or twice daily. It is advisable to consult a healthcare provider for the appropriate dosage and form.

EYEBRIGHT

Overview: Eyebright (Euphrasia officinalis) is a herb traditionally used to treat various eye conditions. It is particularly effective in managing conjunctivitis and other eye irritations due to its anti-inflammatory and astringent properties.

Key Benefits:

- **Treats Conjunctivitis:** Eyebright is commonly used to alleviate symptoms of conjunctivitis (pink eye), such as redness, swelling, and discharge. Its anti-inflammatory properties help reduce inflammation and soothe the eyes.
- **Relieves Eye Irritations:** Eyebright is effective in treating other eye irritations, including blepharitis (inflammation of the eyelids) and styes. It helps to cleanse and soothe irritated eyes.
- **Improves Overall Eye Health:** Regular use of eyebright can help maintain overall eye health by reducing inflammation and preventing infections.

Usage Recommendations:

- **Forms:** Eyebright is available in various forms, including teas, tinctures, eye drops, and capsules.
- **Application:** For treating eye conditions, eyebright can be used as an eye wash or in the form of eye drops. To prepare an eye wash, steep 1-2 teaspoons of dried eyebright in hot water, strain, and allow it to cool. Use the solution to rinse the eyes 2-3 times daily. Eyebright capsules can be taken according to the dosage instructions on the product label or as advised by a healthcare provider.

Considerations:

- **Safety:** Both bilberry and eyebright are generally safe when used as directed. However, individuals with certain medical conditions or those taking specific medications should consult a healthcare provider before use. Bilberry should be used with caution by individuals on blood-thinning medications, and eyebright should be used carefully to avoid contamination if used as an eye wash.
- **Allergic Reactions:** Some people may experience allergic reactions or sensitivity to bilberry or eyebright. It is advisable to perform a patch test (for topical use) and consult a healthcare provider if any adverse effects occur.

Conclusion:

Bilberry and eyebright are effective natural remedies for supporting eye health. Bilberry improves vision and treats eye disorders such as glaucoma and cataracts, while eyebright is beneficial for treating conjunctivitis and other eye irritations. Incorporating these natural remedies into your eye care routine, with appropriate dosages and professional guidance, can help maintain healthy vision and alleviate eye discomfort.

LIVER HEALTH

Maintaining liver health is essential for overall well-being, as the liver plays a crucial role in detoxification, metabolism, and various bodily functions. Natural remedies such as milk thistle and dandelion root have been traditionally used to support liver health and treat liver conditions. These remedies are known for their ability to protect, regenerate, and detoxify the liver.

MILK THISTLE

Overview: Milk thistle (Silybum marianum) is a flowering herb known for its powerful liver-protecting properties. The active compound in milk thistle, silymarin, is renowned for its ability to protect and regenerate liver cells.

Key Benefits:

- **Protects Liver Cells:** Silymarin helps to shield liver cells from damage caused by toxins, alcohol, and other harmful substances. It acts as an antioxidant, neutralizing free radicals and reducing oxidative stress.
- **Regenerates Liver Cells:** Milk thistle promotes the regeneration of new liver cells, helping to repair and rejuvenate the liver.
- **Treats Liver Diseases:** Milk thistle is used to manage and treat various liver conditions, including hepatitis, cirrhosis, and fatty liver disease. It helps to improve liver function and reduce liver enzyme levels.

Usage Recommendations:

- **Forms:** Milk thistle is available in various forms, including capsules, tablets, tinctures, and teas.
- **Dosage:** For liver health, a common dosage is 200-400 mg of milk thistle extract standardized to contain 70-80% silymarin, taken one to three times daily. It is advisable to consult a healthcare provider for the appropriate dosage and form.

DANDELION ROOT

Overview: Dandelion root (Taraxacum officinale) is a traditional herbal remedy known for its role as a liver tonic. It supports liver detoxification and promotes overall liver health.

Key Benefits:

- **Acts as a Liver Tonic:** Dandelion root helps to stimulate bile production, which aids in the digestion and absorption of fats. This promotes liver function and supports the detoxification process.
- **Supports Liver Detoxification:** Dandelion root enhances the liver's ability to filter and remove toxins from the bloodstream, helping to cleanse and purify the liver.
- **Improves Digestion:** By promoting bile flow, dandelion root also aids in digestion and reduces symptoms of indigestion and bloating.

Usage Recommendations:

- **Forms:** Dandelion root is available in various forms, including teas, capsules, tinctures, and extracts.
- **Dosage:** For liver support, a common recommendation is to drink dandelion root tea up to three times daily or take 500-2,000 mg of dandelion root extract in capsule form. Consulting a healthcare provider for specific dosage recommendations is advisable.

Considerations:

- **Safety:** Both milk thistle and dandelion root are generally safe when used as directed. However, individuals with certain medical conditions or those taking specific medications should consult a healthcare provider before use. Milk thistle may interact with medications metabolized by the liver, and dandelion root should be used with caution by individuals with gallbladder issues.

- **Allergic Reactions:** Some people may experience allergic reactions or sensitivity to milk thistle or dandelion root. It is advisable to perform a patch test (for topical use) and consult a healthcare provider if any adverse effects occur.

Conclusion:

Milk thistle and dandelion root are effective natural remedies for supporting liver health. Milk thistle protects and regenerates liver cells, making it beneficial for treating liver diseases and enhancing liver function. Dandelion root acts as a liver tonic and supports detoxification, promoting overall liver health. Incorporating these natural remedies into your liver health routine, with appropriate dosages and professional guidance, can help maintain a healthy liver and improve overall well-being.

KIDNEY HEALTH

Maintaining kidney health is vital for the body's ability to filter waste and regulate fluid balance. Natural remedies such as cranberry and nettle have been traditionally used to support kidney function and prevent urinary tract infections. These remedies are known for their diuretic and antibacterial properties, which help in maintaining healthy kidneys.

CRANBERRY

Overview: Cranberry (Vaccinium macrocarpon) is a fruit commonly used to prevent urinary tract infections (UTIs). It contains compounds that help to prevent bacteria from adhering to the urinary tract walls, thereby reducing the risk of infections.

Key Benefits:

- **Prevents Urinary Tract Infections:** Cranberries contain proanthocyanidins, which inhibit the adhesion of E. coli bacteria to the urinary tract lining, reducing the risk of UTIs.
- **Supports Urinary Health:** Regular consumption of cranberry can help to maintain a healthy urinary tract by reducing the frequency of infections.
- **Antioxidant Properties:** Cranberries are rich in antioxidants, which help to reduce inflammation and protect the cells in the urinary tract from damage.

Usage Recommendations:

- **Forms:** Cranberry is available in various forms, including fresh fruit, juice, capsules, and extracts.
- **Dosage:** For preventing UTIs, a common recommendation is to drink 8-16 ounces of unsweetened cranberry juice daily or take 300-400 mg of cranberry extract in capsule form twice daily. It is advisable to consult a healthcare provider for the appropriate dosage.

NETTLE

Overview: Nettle (Urtica dioica) is a herb known for its diuretic properties and its ability to support kidney function. It helps to promote urine flow and cleanse the kidneys, reducing the risk of kidney stones and other kidney-related issues.

Key Benefits:

- **Acts as a Diuretic:** Nettle increases urine production, which helps to flush out toxins and prevent the formation of kidney stones.
- **Supports Kidney Function:** By promoting urine flow, nettle helps to keep the kidneys clean and functioning efficiently.
- **Reduces Inflammation:** Nettle has anti-inflammatory properties that help to reduce inflammation in the kidneys and urinary tract.

Usage Recommendations:

- **Forms:** Nettle is available in various forms, including teas, capsules, tinctures, and extracts.
- **Dosage:** For kidney health, it is recommended to drink nettle tea up to three times daily or take 300-600 mg of nettle extract in capsule form. Consulting a healthcare provider for specific dosage recommendations is advisable.

Considerations:

- **Safety:** Both cranberry and nettle are generally safe when used as directed. However, individuals with certain medical conditions or those taking specific medications should consult a healthcare provider before use. Cranberry should be used with caution by individuals prone to kidney stones, and nettle may interact with blood-thinning medications.

- **Allergic Reactions:** Some people may experience allergic reactions or gastrointestinal upset when using cranberry or nettle. It is important to monitor your body's response and consult a healthcare provider if any adverse effects occur.

Conclusion:

Cranberry and nettle are effective natural remedies for supporting kidney health. Cranberry helps to prevent urinary tract infections by inhibiting bacterial adhesion to the urinary tract lining. Nettle acts as a diuretic, promoting urine flow and supporting kidney function. Incorporating these natural remedies into your kidney health routine, with appropriate dosages and professional guidance, can help maintain healthy kidneys and prevent urinary tract issues.

RESPIRATORY HEALTH

Maintaining respiratory health is crucial, especially during times of increased exposure to respiratory infections and conditions. Natural remedies such as mullein and oregano oil have been traditionally used to support respiratory function and treat various respiratory conditions. These remedies are known for their anti-inflammatory, antibacterial, and expectorant properties, which help in managing asthma, bronchitis, and respiratory infections.

MULLEIN

Overview: Mullein (Verbascum thapsus) is a plant known for its soothing and healing properties. It has been traditionally used to treat a variety of respiratory conditions, including asthma and bronchitis.

Key Benefits:

- **Treats Asthma and Bronchitis:** Mullein helps to reduce inflammation and relax the muscles in the respiratory tract, making it easier to breathe for individuals with asthma and bronchitis.
- **Expectorant Properties:** Mullein acts as an expectorant, helping to loosen and expel mucus from the respiratory tract. This helps to clear congestion and improve breathing.
- **Soothes Irritated Tissues:** Mullein has demulcent properties, which help to soothe and protect the mucous membranes in the respiratory system, reducing irritation and inflammation.

Usage Recommendations:

- **Forms:** Mullein is available in various forms, including teas, capsules, tinctures, and extracts.
- **Dosage:** For respiratory health, a common recommendation is to drink mullein tea up to three times daily or take 300-500 mg of mullein extract in capsule form. It is advisable to consult a healthcare provider for the appropriate dosage and form.

OREGANO OIL

Overview: Oregano oil (Origanum vulgare) is a potent essential oil known for its antimicrobial properties. It is particularly effective in treating respiratory infections due to its ability to kill bacteria and viruses.

Key Benefits:

- **Clears Respiratory Infections:** Oregano oil contains compounds such as carvacrol and thymol, which have strong antibacterial and antiviral properties. These compounds help to clear respiratory infections and reduce symptoms.
- **Anti-inflammatory Effects:** Oregano oil helps to reduce inflammation in the respiratory tract, making it beneficial for conditions such as asthma, bronchitis, and other inflammatory respiratory diseases.
- **Supports Immune Function:** Oregano oil boosts the immune system, helping the body to fight off infections more effectively and prevent future respiratory issues.

Usage Recommendations:

- **Forms:** Oregano oil is available in various forms, including essential oil, capsules, and liquid extracts.
- **Dosage:** For treating respiratory infections, a common dosage is to take 2-4 drops of oregano oil diluted in water or juice, up to three times daily. Oregano oil capsules can also be taken according to the dosage instructions on the product label. It is important to consult a healthcare provider for specific dosage recommendations and to ensure safe use.

Considerations:

- **Safety:** Both mullein and oregano oil are generally safe when used as directed. However, individuals with certain medical conditions or those taking specific medications should consult a healthcare provider before use. Mullein should be used with caution by individuals with known allergies to plants in the Scrophulariaceae family, and oregano oil should be diluted properly to avoid irritation.
- **Allergic Reactions:** Some people may experience allergic reactions or sensitivity to mullein or oregano oil. It is advisable to perform a patch test (for topical use) and consult a healthcare provider if any adverse effects occur.

Conclusion:

Mullein and oregano oil are effective natural remedies for supporting respiratory health. Mullein helps to treat respiratory conditions such as asthma and bronchitis by reducing inflammation and acting as an expectorant. Oregano oil contains powerful compounds that help to clear respiratory infections and support overall immune function. Incorporating these natural remedies into your respiratory health routine, with appropriate dosages and professional guidance, can help maintain healthy respiratory function and alleviate symptoms of respiratory conditions.

WEIGHT MANAGEMENT

Managing weight effectively is essential for maintaining overall health and preventing chronic diseases. Natural remedies such as green tea and garcinia cambogia have been traditionally used to support weight management. These remedies are known for their ability to boost metabolism, suppress appetite, and prevent fat storage.

GREEN TEA

Overview: Green tea (Camellia sinensis) is widely recognized for its numerous health benefits, including its ability to boost metabolism and aid in weight loss. It contains bioactive compounds such as catechins and caffeine that contribute to its weight management properties.

Key Benefits:

- **Boosts Metabolism:** Green tea increases the rate at which the body burns calories by enhancing thermogenesis, the process of heat production in the body. This helps to increase energy expenditure and promote weight loss.
- **Aids in Fat Burning:** The catechins in green tea, particularly epigallocatechin gallate (EGCG), help to break down fat cells and enhance fat oxidation during exercise.
- **Reduces Appetite:** Green tea can help to reduce appetite and cravings, making it easier to adhere to a calorie-controlled diet.

Usage Recommendations:

- **Forms:** Green tea is available in various forms, including loose leaves, tea bags, capsules, and extracts.
- **Dosage:** For weight management, it is recommended to drink 2-3 cups of green tea daily or take 300-500 mg of green tea extract per day. It is advisable to consult a healthcare provider for the appropriate dosage and form.

GARCINIA CAMBOGIA

Overview: Garcinia cambogia (Garcinia gummi-gutta) is a tropical fruit commonly used in weight loss supplements. Its active ingredient, hydroxycitric acid (HCA), is known for its ability to suppress appetite and prevent fat storage.

Key Benefits:

- **Suppresses Appetite:** Garcinia cambogia increases levels of serotonin in the brain, which can help to reduce appetite and decrease food intake.
- **Prevents Fat Storage:** HCA inhibits an enzyme called citrate lyase, which the body uses to make fat. By blocking this enzyme, garcinia cambogia helps to prevent the storage of fat and reduces the production of new fat cells.
- **Enhances Fat Burning:** Garcinia cambogia can also help to increase fat burning and reduce belly fat, contributing to overall weight loss.

Usage Recommendations:

- **Forms:** Garcinia cambogia is available in various forms, including capsules, tablets, and liquid extracts.
- **Dosage:** For weight management, a common dosage is 500-1,000 mg of garcinia cambogia extract (standardized to contain 50-60% HCA) taken 30-60 minutes before meals, up to three times daily. It is best to consult a healthcare provider for specific dosage recommendations.

Considerations:

- **Safety:** Both green tea and garcinia cambogia are generally safe when used as directed. However, individuals with certain medical conditions or those taking specific medications should consult a healthcare provider before use. Green tea contains caffeine, which can cause jitteriness and sleep disturbances in sensitive individuals. Garcinia cambogia should be used with caution by individuals with liver conditions or those taking medications that affect serotonin levels.

- **Side Effects:** Some people may experience side effects such as digestive upset, headache, or dizziness. It is important to monitor your body's response and consult a healthcare provider if any adverse effects occur.

Conclusion:

Green tea and garcinia cambogia are effective natural remedies for supporting weight management. Green tea boosts metabolism and aids in fat burning, while garcinia cambogia suppresses appetite and prevents fat storage. Incorporating these natural remedies into your weight management routine, with appropriate dosages and professional guidance, can help you achieve and maintain a healthy weight.

SLEEP DISORDERS

Effectively managing sleep disorders is crucial for overall health and well-being. Natural remedies such as passionflower and hops have been traditionally used to improve sleep quality and treat conditions like insomnia and anxiety. These remedies are known for their calming and sedative properties, which help promote restful sleep.

PASSIONFLOWER

Overview: Passionflower (Passiflora incarnata) is an herb that has been used for centuries to treat insomnia and anxiety. It works by increasing levels of gamma-aminobutyric acid (GABA) in the brain, which helps to calm the mind and promote relaxation.

Key Benefits:

- **Treats Insomnia:** Passionflower is effective in helping individuals fall asleep faster and improving the overall quality of sleep. It is particularly beneficial for those who have difficulty staying asleep.
- **Reduces Anxiety:** By increasing GABA levels, passionflower helps to reduce anxiety and nervousness, making it easier to relax and fall asleep.
- **Promotes Relaxation:** The calming effects of passionflower help to ease the mind and body, reducing restlessness and promoting a state of relaxation conducive to sleep.

Usage Recommendations:

- **Forms:** Passionflower is available in various forms, including teas, capsules, tinctures, and extracts.
- **Dosage:** For treating insomnia and anxiety, a common recommendation is to drink passionflower tea up to three times daily or take 300-500 mg of passionflower extract in capsule form. It is advisable to consult a healthcare provider for the appropriate dosage and form.

HOPS

Overview: Hops (Humulus lupulus) are commonly known for their use in brewing beer, but they also have medicinal properties that can improve sleep quality. Hops are often used in combination with valerian root to enhance their sedative effects.

Key Benefits:

- **Improves Sleep Quality:** Hops help to improve sleep quality by promoting relaxation and reducing the time it takes to fall asleep. They have a mild sedative effect that makes them effective for treating sleep disorders.
- **Reduces Anxiety:** Hops have calming properties that help to reduce anxiety and stress, which can contribute to better sleep.
- **Enhances Valerian Root Effects:** When used in combination with valerian root, hops can enhance the sedative effects, making the combination more effective for improving sleep quality.

Usage Recommendations:

- **Forms:** Hops are available in various forms, including teas, capsules, tinctures, and extracts. They are often combined with valerian root in sleep aid supplements.
- **Dosage:** For improving sleep quality, a common recommendation is to take a combination of 300-600 mg of valerian root and 30-120 mg of hops extract before bedtime. It is best to consult a healthcare provider for specific dosage recommendations.

Considerations:

- **Safety:** Both passionflower and hops are generally safe when used as directed. However, individuals with certain medical conditions or those taking specific medications should consult a healthcare provider before use. Passionflower may interact with sedatives and blood-thinning medications, and hops should be used with caution by individuals with hormone-sensitive conditions.
- **Side Effects:** Some people may experience side effects such as dizziness, digestive upset, or allergic reactions. It is important to monitor your body's response and consult a healthcare provider if any adverse effects occur.

Conclusion:

Passionflower and hops are effective natural remedies for managing sleep disorders and improving sleep quality. Passionflower helps to treat insomnia and reduce anxiety by promoting relaxation and increasing GABA levels. Hops, particularly when used in combination with valerian root, enhance sleep quality by promoting relaxation and reducing the time it takes to fall asleep. Incorporating these natural remedies into your sleep routine, with appropriate dosages and professional guidance, can help you achieve restful and restorative sleep.

SEXUAL HEALTH

Maintaining sexual health is vital for overall well-being and quality of life. Natural remedies such as maca root and tribulus terrestris have been traditionally used to enhance libido, sexual function, and performance. These remedies are known for their ability to boost sexual desire and improve reproductive health.

MACA ROOT

Overview: Maca root (Lepidium meyenii) is a root vegetable native to the Andes of Peru, often referred to as a superfood due to its rich nutritional profile. It is widely recognized for its ability to enhance libido and sexual function in both men and women.

Key Benefits:

- **Enhances Libido:** Maca root has been shown to increase sexual desire in both men and women. It works by balancing hormone levels and supporting overall sexual health.
- **Improves Sexual Function:** Regular use of maca root can improve sexual performance, including erectile function in men and overall sexual satisfaction in women.
- **Supports Reproductive Health:** Maca root is also beneficial for reproductive health, improving sperm quality in men and balancing menstrual cycles in women.

Usage Recommendations:

- **Forms:** Maca root is available in various forms, including powder, capsules, and extracts. The powder can be easily added to smoothies, oatmeal, or other foods.
- **Dosage:** For enhancing libido and sexual function, a common dosage is 1,500-3,000 mg of maca root powder daily. It is advisable to consult a healthcare provider for the appropriate dosage based on individual health needs.

TRIBULUS TERRESTRIS

Overview: Tribulus terrestris is a plant used in traditional medicine to improve sexual desire and performance. It is known for its ability to enhance libido, increase testosterone levels, and support overall sexual health.

Key Benefits:

- **Improves Sexual Desire:** Tribulus terrestris helps to boost libido by increasing the production of sex hormones, such as testosterone, which are essential for sexual desire.
- **Enhances Sexual Performance:** This herb is effective in improving sexual performance, including erectile function in men and sexual satisfaction in women.
- **Supports Hormonal Balance:** Tribulus terrestris helps to balance hormones, which can enhance reproductive health and overall sexual function.

Usage Recommendations:

- **Forms:** Tribulus terrestris is available in various forms, including capsules, tablets, and extracts.
- **Dosage:** For improving sexual desire and performance, a common dosage is 500-1,500 mg of tribulus terrestris extract daily. It is best to consult a healthcare provider for specific dosage recommendations based on individual health needs.

Considerations:

- **Safety:** Both maca root and tribulus terrestris are generally safe when used as directed. However, individuals with certain medical conditions or those taking specific medications should consult a healthcare provider before use. Maca root should be used with caution by individuals with thyroid issues, and tribulus terrestris should be avoided by individuals with hormone-sensitive conditions.
- **Side Effects:** Some people may experience side effects such as digestive upset, headache, or skin reactions. It is important to monitor your body's response and consult a healthcare provider if any adverse effects occur.

Conclusion:

Maca root and tribulus terrestris are effective natural remedies for enhancing sexual health. Maca root boosts libido and sexual function by balancing hormones and supporting reproductive health, while tribulus terrestris improves sexual desire and performance by increasing testosterone levels and enhancing hormonal balance. Incorporating these natural remedies into your health routine, with appropriate dosages and professional guidance, can help you achieve better sexual health and overall well-being.

HAIR HEALTH

Maintaining healthy hair is essential for overall appearance and confidence. Natural remedies such as rosemary and horsetail have been traditionally used to promote hair growth, treat dandruff, and strengthen hair. These remedies are known for their beneficial properties that support and enhance hair health.

ROSEMARY

Overview: Rosemary (Rosmarinus officinalis) is an herb commonly used in cooking and traditional medicine. It is well-known for its ability to stimulate hair growth and treat dandruff.

Key Benefits:

- **Stimulates Hair Growth:** Rosemary improves blood circulation to the scalp, which helps to nourish hair follicles and promote hair growth. It has been shown to increase hair count and thickness.
- **Treats Dandruff:** Rosemary has antifungal and antibacterial properties that help to combat dandruff and soothe an itchy scalp. It helps to reduce flakiness and maintain a healthy scalp environment.
- **Strengthens Hair:** The antioxidant properties of rosemary help to strengthen hair and protect it from damage caused by free radicals and environmental stressors.

Usage Recommendations:

- **Forms:** Rosemary can be used as an essential oil, in hair rinses, or infused in shampoos and conditioners.
- **Application:** For hair growth and dandruff treatment, mix a few drops of rosemary essential oil with a carrier oil (such as coconut or olive oil) and massage into the scalp. Leave it on for at least 30 minutes before washing it out. This can be done 1-2 times per week.

HORSETAIL

Overview: Horsetail (Equisetum arvense) is a plant known for its high silica content, which is essential for healthy hair and nails. It has been used for centuries to strengthen hair and promote overall hair health.

Key Benefits:

- **Rich in Silica:** Horsetail is one of the richest plant sources of silica, a mineral that helps to strengthen hair and nails. Silica improves hair texture, reduces brittleness, and enhances shine.
- **Strengthens Hair:** The nutrients in horsetail help to strengthen hair from the roots, reducing hair breakage and promoting healthier, thicker hair.
- **Improves Scalp Health:** Horsetail has anti-inflammatory and antimicrobial properties that help to maintain a healthy scalp, which is crucial for healthy hair growth.

Usage Recommendations:

- **Forms:** Horsetail is available in various forms, including capsules, teas, and extracts.
- **Dosage:** For hair health, a common dosage is 300-500 mg of horsetail extract in capsule form daily, or drinking horsetail tea up to twice daily. It is advisable to consult a healthcare provider for the appropriate dosage and form.

Considerations:

- **Safety:** Both rosemary and horsetail are generally safe when used as directed. However, individuals with certain medical conditions or those taking specific medications should consult a healthcare provider before use. Rosemary essential oil should not be ingested and should be used with caution in individuals with epilepsy or hypertension. Horsetail should be used with caution by individuals with kidney issues due to its diuretic properties.

- **Allergic Reactions:** Some people may experience allergic reactions or skin irritation when using rosemary or horsetail. It is advisable to perform a patch test (for topical use) and consult a healthcare provider if any adverse effects occur.

Conclusion:

Rosemary and horsetail are effective natural remedies for supporting and enhancing hair health. Rosemary stimulates hair growth and treats dandruff by improving scalp health and circulation. Horsetail, rich in silica, strengthens hair and nails, reducing brittleness and promoting healthier hair. Incorporating these natural remedies into your hair care routine, with appropriate applications and professional guidance, can help you achieve stronger, healthier, and more vibrant hair.

BONE AND JOINT HEALTH

Maintaining bone and joint health is crucial for mobility and overall quality of life. Natural remedies such as boswellia and hyaluronic acid have been traditionally used to reduce inflammation, treat arthritis, and support joint health. These remedies are known for their anti-inflammatory properties and ability to improve joint function and comfort.

BOSWELLIA

Overview: Boswellia (Boswellia serrata), also known as Indian frankincense, is a resin extracted from the boswellia tree. It is widely used in traditional medicine to treat inflammation and arthritis.

Key Benefits:

- **Reduces Inflammation:** Boswellia contains active compounds called boswellic acids, which have strong anti-inflammatory effects. These compounds inhibit inflammatory pathways, reducing swelling and pain in the joints.
- **Treats Arthritis:** Boswellia is particularly effective in treating osteoarthritis and rheumatoid arthritis. It helps to improve joint function and reduce symptoms such as pain, stiffness, and loss of mobility.
- **Promotes Joint Health:** By reducing inflammation and pain, boswellia supports overall joint health and helps prevent further damage to the cartilage and joint tissues.

Usage Recommendations:

- **Forms:** Boswellia is available in various forms, including capsules, tablets, and topical creams.
- **Dosage:** For treating arthritis and inflammation, a common dosage is 300-500 mg of boswellia extract standardized to contain 60-70% boswellic acids, taken two to three times daily. It is advisable to consult a healthcare provider for the appropriate dosage and form.

HYALURONIC ACID

Overview: Hyaluronic acid is a naturally occurring substance in the body that plays a key role in maintaining joint lubrication and health. It is commonly used to treat arthritis and support joint function.

Key Benefits:

- **Supports Joint Lubrication:** Hyaluronic acid helps to maintain the synovial fluid that lubricates joints, reducing friction and allowing for smooth, pain-free movement.
- **Reduces Arthritis Symptoms:** Hyaluronic acid injections or supplements can help to reduce symptoms of arthritis, such as pain, stiffness, and swelling. It helps to improve joint function and mobility.
- **Promotes Joint Health:** By providing lubrication and cushioning, hyaluronic acid helps to protect joints from wear and tear, supporting overall joint health and longevity.

Usage Recommendations:

- **Forms:** Hyaluronic acid is available in various forms, including oral supplements, topical creams, and injectable treatments.
- **Dosage:** For joint health, a common oral dosage is 50-200 mg of hyaluronic acid per day. Injectable treatments should be administered by a healthcare professional. It is advisable to consult a healthcare provider for the appropriate dosage and form.

Considerations:

- **Safety:** Both boswellia and hyaluronic acid are generally safe when used as directed. However, individuals with certain medical conditions or those taking specific medications should consult a healthcare provider before use. Boswellia may interact with medications that affect the liver, and hyaluronic acid injections should be administered by a healthcare professional to avoid complications.

- **Side Effects:** Some people may experience side effects such as digestive upset or allergic reactions with boswellia. Hyaluronic acid supplements are generally well-tolerated, but injections may cause temporary pain or swelling at the injection site. It is important to monitor your body's response and consult a healthcare provider if any adverse effects occur.

Conclusion:

Boswellia and hyaluronic acid are effective natural remedies for supporting bone and joint health. Boswellia reduces inflammation and treats arthritis by inhibiting inflammatory pathways and improving joint function. Hyaluronic acid supports joint lubrication and reduces arthritis symptoms by maintaining synovial fluid and protecting joints. Incorporating these natural remedies into your health routine, with appropriate dosages and professional guidance, can help you achieve better joint health and reduce the symptoms of arthritis.

DETOXIFICATION

Effective detoxification is crucial for maintaining overall health and well-being, as it helps to remove toxins and impurities from the body. Natural remedies such as burdock root and chlorella have been traditionally used to support detoxification processes. These remedies are known for their ability to purify the blood, support liver function, and aid in the removal of heavy metals and toxins.

BURDOCK ROOT

Overview: Burdock root (Arctium lappa) is a vegetable with a long history of use in traditional medicine. It is known for its powerful detoxifying properties and its ability to purify the blood and support liver function.

Key Benefits:

- **Purifies the Blood:** Burdock root helps to eliminate toxins from the bloodstream, enhancing the body's natural detoxification processes. It is particularly effective in promoting healthy skin by reducing impurities that can cause skin issues.
- **Supports Liver Detoxification:** Burdock root stimulates bile production and supports liver function, helping to detoxify the liver and improve its ability to process and eliminate toxins.
- **Anti-inflammatory Properties:** Burdock root has anti-inflammatory effects that can help reduce inflammation throughout the body, promoting overall health and well-being.

Usage Recommendations:

- **Forms:** Burdock root is available in various forms, including fresh root, dried root, capsules, tinctures, and teas.
- **Dosage:** For detoxification, a common recommendation is to drink burdock root tea up to three times daily or take 300-500 mg of burdock root extract in capsule form. It is advisable to consult a healthcare provider for the appropriate dosage and form.

CHLORELLA

Overview: Chlorella is a type of freshwater algae known for its powerful detoxifying abilities. It is particularly effective in binding to heavy metals and other toxins, aiding in their removal from the body.

Key Benefits:

- **Binds to Heavy Metals:** Chlorella contains chlorophyll and other compounds that bind to heavy metals, such as mercury, cadmium, and lead, helping to detoxify the body by facilitating their removal.
- **Aids in Toxin Removal:** Chlorella supports the elimination of toxins from the body by enhancing liver function and promoting regular bowel movements.
- **Nutrient-Rich:** In addition to its detoxifying properties, chlorella is rich in vitamins, minerals, and antioxidants, which support overall health and boost the immune system.

Usage Recommendations:

- **Forms:** Chlorella is available in various forms, including tablets, capsules, powders, and extracts.
- **Dosage:** For detoxification, a common dosage is 2-4 grams of chlorella per day, taken with water or juice. It is best to start with a lower dose and gradually increase to avoid digestive discomfort. Consulting a healthcare provider for specific dosage recommendations is advisable.

Considerations:

- **Safety:** Both burdock root and chlorella are generally safe when used as directed. However, individuals with certain medical conditions or those taking specific medications should consult a healthcare provider before use. Burdock root should be used with caution by individuals with allergies to plants in the Asteraceae family, and chlorella may cause digestive upset in some individuals.

- **Allergic Reactions:** Some people may experience allergic reactions or sensitivity to burdock root or chlorella. It is advisable to perform a patch test (for topical use) and consult a healthcare provider if any adverse effects occur.

Conclusion:

Burdock root and chlorella are effective natural remedies for supporting detoxification. Burdock root purifies the blood and supports liver detoxification by enhancing bile production and eliminating toxins. Chlorella binds to heavy metals and toxins, aiding in their removal from the body and supporting overall detoxification processes. Incorporating these natural remedies into your detox routine, with appropriate dosages and professional guidance, can help maintain a clean, toxin-free system and promote overall health.

ALLERGIES

Managing allergies effectively is essential for maintaining comfort and overall well-being, especially during allergy seasons. Natural remedies such as butterbur and quercetin have been traditionally used to alleviate allergy symptoms. These remedies are known for their ability to reduce the severity of allergic reactions and act as natural antihistamines.

BUTTERBUR

Overview: Butterbur (Petasites hybridus) is a plant traditionally used for its anti-inflammatory and anti-allergic properties. It is particularly effective in reducing the severity of allergic reactions, especially those associated with hay fever.

Key Benefits:

- **Reduces Allergy Symptoms:** Butterbur helps to alleviate common allergy symptoms such as sneezing, nasal congestion, and itchy eyes. It works by inhibiting the production of histamines and leukotrienes, which are chemicals involved in the allergic response.
- **Anti-inflammatory Properties:** Butterbur reduces inflammation in the respiratory tract, helping to ease symptoms of allergic rhinitis and other respiratory allergies.
- **Non-Drowsy Alternative:** Unlike many over-the-counter antihistamines, butterbur does not typically cause drowsiness, making it a preferable option for daytime use.

Usage Recommendations:

- **Forms:** Butterbur is available in various forms, including capsules, tablets, and extracts. It is important to choose products labeled as PA-free (pyrrolizidine alkaloids-free) to ensure safety.
- **Dosage:** For allergy relief, a common dosage is 50-75 mg of butterbur extract taken twice daily. It is advisable to consult a healthcare provider for the appropriate dosage and form.

QUERCETIN

Overview: Quercetin is a natural flavonoid found in many fruits and vegetables, such as apples, onions, and berries. It is known for its potent antioxidant and anti-inflammatory properties, as well as its ability to act as a natural antihistamine.

Key Benefits:

- **Natural Antihistamine:** Quercetin stabilizes mast cells, which release histamines during allergic reactions. By reducing histamine release, quercetin helps to alleviate symptoms such as sneezing, itching, and nasal congestion.
- **Reduces Inflammation:** Quercetin's anti-inflammatory properties help to reduce inflammation in the respiratory tract, making it beneficial for managing symptoms of allergic rhinitis and asthma.
- **Supports Immune Health:** Quercetin boosts the immune system and helps to protect cells from oxidative stress, supporting overall health and resilience against allergens.

Usage Recommendations:

- **Forms:** Quercetin is available in various forms, including capsules, tablets, and powders. It is also present in significant amounts in certain foods.
- **Dosage:** For allergy relief, a common dosage is 500-1,000 mg of quercetin daily, divided into two or three doses. It is best to start with a lower dose and gradually increase to avoid digestive discomfort. Consulting a healthcare provider for specific dosage recommendations is advisable.

Considerations:

- **Safety:** Both butterbur and quercetin are generally safe when used as directed. However, individuals with certain medical conditions or those taking specific medications should consult a healthcare provider before use. Butterbur should be PA-free to avoid potential liver toxicity, and quercetin should be used with caution by individuals with kidney issues.
- **Allergic Reactions:** Some people may experience allergic reactions or sensitivity to butterbur or quercetin. It is advisable to perform a patch test (for topical use) and consult a healthcare provider if any adverse effects occur.

Conclusion:

Butterbur and quercetin are effective natural remedies for managing allergies. Butterbur reduces the severity of allergic reactions by inhibiting histamine and leukotriene production, while quercetin acts as a natural antihistamine and reduces inflammation. Incorporating these natural remedies into your allergy management routine, with appropriate dosages and professional guidance, can help alleviate symptoms and improve overall comfort during allergy seasons.

HORMONAL BALANCE

Maintaining hormonal balance is essential for overall health and well-being, as hormones regulate many critical bodily functions. Natural remedies such as ashwagandha and rhodiola have been traditionally used to support hormonal health. These remedies are known for their ability to reduce stress, balance cortisol levels, and support adrenal function.

ASHWAGANDHA

Overview: Ashwagandha (Withania somnifera) is a powerful adaptogen that has been used in Ayurvedic medicine for centuries. It is well-known for its ability to support adrenal health and balance hormones.

Key Benefits:

- **Supports Adrenal Health:** Ashwagandha helps to nourish and support the adrenal glands, which are responsible for producing hormones such as cortisol and adrenaline. This support helps to maintain balanced hormone levels and reduce adrenal fatigue.
- **Balances Hormones:** By modulating the endocrine system, ashwagandha helps to balance hormones, including thyroid hormones, cortisol, and reproductive hormones. This can improve overall hormonal health and reduce symptoms of hormonal imbalances.
- **Reduces Stress and Anxiety:** Ashwagandha lowers cortisol levels, which can help to reduce stress and anxiety. Lower cortisol levels also contribute to improved mood and overall mental well-being.

Usage Recommendations:

- **Forms:** Ashwagandha is available in various forms, including capsules, powders, and tinctures.
- **Dosage:** For hormonal balance, a common dosage is 300-600 mg of ashwagandha extract taken once or twice daily. It is advisable to consult a healthcare provider for the appropriate dosage and form based on individual health needs.

RHODIOLA

Overview: Rhodiola (Rhodiola rosea) is another potent adaptogen known for its ability to reduce stress and balance cortisol levels. It has been used in traditional medicine to enhance physical and mental performance and support overall health.

Key Benefits:

- **Reduces Stress:** Rhodiola helps the body adapt to stress by balancing cortisol levels, the hormone released during stressful situations. By reducing cortisol levels, rhodiola helps to alleviate stress and improve resilience.
- **Balances Cortisol Levels:** Rhodiola regulates cortisol production, ensuring that cortisol levels remain balanced. This helps to prevent the negative effects of high cortisol, such as weight gain, fatigue, and impaired immune function.
- **Improves Mood and Cognitive Function:** Rhodiola has been shown to enhance mood, reduce symptoms of depression, and improve cognitive function. This contributes to better overall mental health and well-being.

Usage Recommendations:

- **Forms:** Rhodiola is available in various forms, including capsules, tablets, and tinctures.
- **Dosage:** For balancing cortisol levels and reducing stress, a common dosage is 200-400 mg of rhodiola extract taken once or twice daily. It is best to start with a lower dose and gradually increase as needed. Consulting a healthcare provider for specific dosage recommendations is advisable.

Considerations:

- **Safety:** Both ashwagandha and rhodiola are generally safe when used as directed. However, individuals with certain medical conditions or those taking specific medications should consult a healthcare provider before use. Ashwagandha should be used with caution by individuals with thyroid disorders, and rhodiola may interact with antidepressants and other medications.
- **Side Effects:** Some people may experience side effects such as digestive upset, headache, or dizziness. It is important to monitor your body's response and consult a healthcare provider if any adverse effects occur.

Conclusion:

Ashwagandha and rhodiola are effective natural remedies for supporting hormonal balance. Ashwagandha supports adrenal health and balances hormones by modulating the endocrine system and reducing cortisol levels. Rhodiola reduces stress and balances cortisol levels, improving mood and cognitive function. Incorporating these natural remedies into your health routine, with appropriate dosages and professional guidance, can help maintain balanced hormones and enhance overall well-being.

INFLAMMATION

Effectively managing inflammation is crucial for overall health and can help prevent chronic diseases. Natural remedies such as turmeric and bromelain have been traditionally used to reduce inflammation and alleviate related symptoms. These remedies are known for their potent anti-inflammatory properties.

TURMERIC

Overview: Turmeric (Curcuma longa) is a spice commonly used in cooking and traditional medicine. Its active ingredient, curcumin, is renowned for its powerful anti-inflammatory and antioxidant effects.

Key Benefits:

- **Reduces Inflammation:** Curcumin inhibits inflammatory pathways in the body, reducing inflammation and associated pain. It is particularly beneficial for conditions such as arthritis, where inflammation is a major symptom.
- **Antioxidant Properties:** Curcumin is a potent antioxidant, helping to neutralize free radicals and reduce oxidative stress. This not only aids in inflammation reduction but also promotes overall health by protecting cells from damage.
- **Supports Joint Health:** Regular use of turmeric can improve joint function and reduce symptoms of joint-related conditions such as osteoarthritis and rheumatoid arthritis.

Usage Recommendations:

- **Forms:** Turmeric can be consumed as a spice in food, in supplements, or as a tea. For enhanced absorption, it is often combined with black pepper, which contains piperine, a compound that increases curcumin's bioavailability.
- **Dosage:** For reducing inflammation, a common dosage is 500-2,000 mg of turmeric extract per day, standardized to contain 95% curcuminoids. It is advisable to consult a

healthcare provider for the appropriate dosage.

BROMELAIN

Overview: Bromelain is an enzyme found in pineapple (Ananas comosus). It is known for its ability to reduce inflammation and swelling, making it a popular natural remedy for various inflammatory conditions.

Key Benefits:

- **Reduces Inflammation and Swelling:** Bromelain helps to break down proteins that cause inflammation and swelling in the body. It is particularly effective in reducing symptoms of sinusitis, arthritis, and other inflammatory conditions.
- **Supports Digestive Health:** Bromelain aids in the digestion of proteins, promoting better digestive health and reducing inflammation in the digestive tract.
- **Enhances Recovery:** Bromelain is often used to reduce inflammation and speed up recovery after surgeries or injuries, thanks to its ability to minimize swelling and bruising.

Usage Recommendations:

- **Forms:** Bromelain is available in various forms, including fresh pineapple, supplements, and extracts.
- **Dosage:** For reducing inflammation, a common dosage is 200-800 mg of bromelain per day, taken in divided doses between meals. It is advisable to consult a healthcare provider for the appropriate dosage and form.

Considerations:

- **Safety:** Both turmeric and bromelain are generally safe when used as directed. However, individuals with certain medical conditions or those taking specific medications should consult a healthcare provider before use. Turmeric may interact with blood thinners, and bromelain should be used with caution by individuals with allergies to pineapple or those taking anticoagulants.

- **Side Effects:** Some people may experience side effects such as digestive upset or allergic reactions. It is important to monitor your body's response and consult a healthcare provider if any adverse effects occur.

Conclusion:

Turmeric and bromelain are effective natural remedies for managing inflammation. Turmeric, with its potent anti-inflammatory and antioxidant properties, is particularly beneficial for reducing inflammation and pain associated with conditions such as arthritis. Bromelain, found in pineapple, helps to reduce inflammation and swelling, supporting recovery from injuries and improving digestive health. Incorporating these natural remedies into your health routine, with appropriate dosages and professional guidance, can help reduce inflammation and enhance overall well-being.

BLOOD SUGAR REGULATION

Regulating blood sugar levels is essential for preventing and managing diabetes and maintaining overall health. Natural remedies such as cinnamon and Gymnema sylvestre have been traditionally used to help control blood sugar levels. These remedies are known for their ability to lower blood sugar, reduce sugar absorption, and curb sugar cravings.

CINNAMON

Overview: Cinnamon (Cinnamomum spp.) is a widely used spice known for its medicinal properties, particularly its ability to help lower blood sugar levels.

Key Benefits:

- **Lowers Blood Sugar Levels:** Cinnamon improves insulin sensitivity, allowing cells to use glucose more effectively. This helps to lower blood sugar levels and manage insulin resistance.
- **Reduces Fasting Blood Glucose:** Regular consumption of cinnamon can help reduce fasting blood glucose levels, making it beneficial for individuals with type 2 diabetes.
- **Antioxidant Properties:** Cinnamon contains powerful antioxidants that help to reduce oxidative stress and inflammation, which can contribute to better overall health and improved blood sugar control.

Usage Recommendations:

- **Forms:** Cinnamon is available in various forms, including ground spice, sticks, capsules, and extracts. Ceylon cinnamon is often recommended over cassia cinnamon due to its lower coumarin content.
- **Dosage:** For blood sugar regulation, a common dosage is 1-6 grams of ground cinnamon per day, or 250-500 mg of cinnamon extract taken twice daily. It is advisable to consult a healthcare provider for the appropriate dosage and form.

GYMNEMA SYLVESTRE

Overview: Gymnema sylvestre is an herb traditionally used in Ayurvedic medicine to support blood sugar control. It is known for its ability to reduce sugar absorption and cravings.

Key Benefits:

- **Reduces Sugar Absorption:** Gymnema sylvestre contains compounds called gymnemic acids that block the absorption of sugar in the intestines, helping to lower blood sugar levels.
- **Curbs Sugar Cravings:** Gymnema sylvestre can reduce the taste of sweetness, making sugary foods less appealing and helping to curb sugar cravings. This can be beneficial for weight management and blood sugar control.
- **Supports Insulin Function:** Gymnema sylvestre helps to improve insulin function and enhance glucose uptake by cells, which aids in regulating blood sugar levels.

Usage Recommendations:

- **Forms:** Gymnema sylvestre is available in various forms, including capsules, tablets, powders, and teas.
- **Dosage:** For blood sugar regulation, a common dosage is 200-400 mg of Gymnema sylvestre extract taken twice daily. It is advisable to consult a healthcare provider for the appropriate dosage and form.

Considerations:

- **Safety:** Both cinnamon and Gymnema sylvestre are generally safe when used as directed. However, individuals with certain medical conditions or those taking specific medications should consult a healthcare provider before use. Cinnamon, particularly cassia cinnamon, should be used with caution by individuals with liver conditions due to its coumarin content. Gymnema sylvestre should be used with caution by individuals with hypoglycemia or those taking medications that lower blood sugar.

- **Side Effects:** Some people may experience side effects such as digestive upset or allergic reactions. It is important to monitor your body's response and consult a healthcare provider if any adverse effects occur.

Conclusion:

Cinnamon and Gymnema sylvestre are effective natural remedies for supporting blood sugar regulation. Cinnamon helps to lower blood sugar levels and improve insulin sensitivity, while Gymnema sylvestre reduces sugar absorption and curbs sugar cravings. Incorporating these natural remedies into your health routine, with appropriate dosages and professional guidance, can help maintain stable blood sugar levels and support overall metabolic health.

URINARY HEALTH

Maintaining urinary health is crucial for preventing infections and ensuring the proper functioning of the urinary system. Natural remedies such as D-mannose and corn silk have been traditionally used to support urinary health. These remedies are known for their ability to prevent urinary tract infections (UTIs) and soothe the urinary tract.

D-MANNOSE

Overview: D-mannose is a type of sugar related to glucose, commonly found in fruits like cranberries. It is particularly effective in preventing and treating urinary tract infections (UTIs) by preventing bacteria from adhering to the walls of the urinary tract.

Key Benefits:

- **Prevents UTIs:** D-mannose prevents bacteria, especially E. coli, from sticking to the lining of the urinary tract. This helps to flush out the bacteria during urination, reducing the risk of infection.
- **Treats UTIs:** Regular intake of D-mannose can help to treat existing UTIs by promoting the removal of bacteria from the urinary tract, alleviating symptoms and speeding up recovery.
- **Non-Antibiotic Treatment:** D-mannose offers a natural alternative to antibiotics for managing UTIs, which can be beneficial for individuals who are resistant to antibiotics or wish to avoid their side effects.

Usage Recommendations:

- **Forms:** D-mannose is available in various forms, including powder, capsules, and tablets.
- **Dosage:** For preventing UTIs, a common dosage is 500-2,000 mg of D-mannose per day. For treating an existing UTI, higher doses of 2,000-3,000 mg taken every few hours are often recommended. It is advisable to consult a healthcare provider for the appropriate dosage based on individual needs.

CORN SILK

Overview: Corn silk (Zea mays) is the long, thread-like strands found under the husk of corn. It has been traditionally used as a natural remedy for various urinary conditions due to its soothing and diuretic properties.

Key Benefits:

- **Acts as a Diuretic:** Corn silk helps to increase urine production, promoting the flushing out of toxins and bacteria from the urinary tract. This diuretic effect can help prevent and manage urinary tract infections.
- **Soothes the Urinary Tract:** Corn silk contains compounds that soothe inflammation and irritation in the urinary tract, providing relief from symptoms such as burning and discomfort during urination.
- **Supports Kidney Health:** By promoting urine flow and reducing inflammation, corn silk supports overall kidney health and helps to prevent the formation of kidney stones.

Usage Recommendations:

- **Forms:** Corn silk is available in various forms, including dried corn silk, teas, capsules, and tinctures.
- **Dosage:** For urinary health, a common recommendation is to drink corn silk tea up to three times daily or take 400-450 mg of corn silk extract in capsule form. Consulting a healthcare provider for specific dosage recommendations is advisable.

Considerations:

- **Safety:** Both D-mannose and corn silk are generally safe when used as directed. However, individuals with certain medical conditions or those taking specific medications should consult a healthcare provider before use. D-mannose should be used with caution by individuals with diabetes due to its sugar content, and corn silk should be used cautiously by those with low potassium levels or taking diuretic medications.

- **Allergic Reactions:** Some people may experience allergic reactions or sensitivity to D-mannose or corn silk. It is important to monitor your body's response and consult a healthcare provider if any adverse effects occur.

Conclusion:

D-mannose and corn silk are effective natural remedies for supporting urinary health. D-mannose helps to prevent and treat urinary tract infections by preventing bacterial adhesion to the urinary tract lining. Corn silk acts as a diuretic and soothes the urinary tract, promoting overall urinary health and reducing symptoms of irritation. Incorporating these natural remedies into your urinary health routine, with appropriate dosages and professional guidance, can help maintain a healthy urinary system and prevent infections.

WOUND HEALING

Proper wound healing is essential for preventing infections and promoting recovery. Natural remedies such as honey and gotu kola have been traditionally used to aid in the healing process. These remedies are known for their antibacterial properties and ability to promote tissue repair and reduce scarring.

HONEY

Overview: Honey, particularly medical-grade honey like Manuka honey, has been used for centuries for its medicinal properties. It is renowned for its antibacterial, anti-inflammatory, and healing properties.

Key Benefits:

- **Antibacterial Properties:** Honey's high sugar content and low pH create an environment that inhibits the growth of bacteria. It also contains hydrogen peroxide, which further contributes to its antibacterial effects.
- **Promotes Wound Healing:** Honey helps to keep the wound moist and provides a protective barrier, which supports the natural healing process. It can help to accelerate tissue regeneration and reduce healing time.
- **Reduces Inflammation:** Honey has anti-inflammatory properties that help to reduce swelling, pain, and redness in the wound area.

Usage Recommendations:

- **Forms:** Honey can be applied directly to wounds in its raw form or as medical-grade honey products like Manuka honey.
- **Application:** For wound healing, clean the wound thoroughly and apply a thin layer of honey directly to the affected area. Cover with a sterile bandage and change the dressing as needed, typically once or twice daily. It is advisable to consult a healthcare provider for severe wounds or burns.

GOTU KOLA

Overview: Gotu kola (Centella asiatica) is an herb traditionally used in Ayurvedic and Chinese medicine. It is known for its ability to promote wound healing and reduce scarring.

Key Benefits:

- **Promotes Wound Healing:** Gotu kola stimulates the production of collagen, which is essential for wound healing and tissue repair. It helps to strengthen the skin and promote faster healing.
- **Reduces Scarring:** By enhancing collagen synthesis, gotu kola helps to improve the texture and appearance of scars, making them less noticeable.
- **Anti-inflammatory Properties:** Gotu kola reduces inflammation in the wound area, helping to alleviate pain and swelling.

Usage Recommendations:

- **Forms:** Gotu kola is available in various forms, including creams, ointments, capsules, and extracts.
- **Application:** For topical use, apply gotu kola cream or ointment directly to the wound area 2-3 times daily. For internal use, a common dosage is 500-1,000 mg of gotu kola extract in capsule form, taken daily. It is advisable to consult a healthcare provider for the appropriate form and dosage.

Considerations:

- **Safety:** Both honey and gotu kola are generally safe when used as directed. However, individuals with certain medical conditions or those taking specific medications should consult a healthcare provider before use. Honey should not be used on infants under one year of age due to the risk of botulism, and individuals allergic to bee products should avoid using honey. Gotu kola should be used with caution by individuals with liver conditions.

- **Allergic Reactions:** Some people may experience allergic reactions or sensitivity to honey or gotu kola. It is important to monitor your body's response and consult a healthcare provider if any adverse effects occur.

Conclusion:

Honey and gotu kola are effective natural remedies for promoting wound healing. Honey's antibacterial properties help to prevent infection and accelerate healing, while gotu kola promotes tissue repair and reduces scarring. Incorporating these natural remedies into your wound care routine, with appropriate applications and professional guidance, can help ensure proper wound healing and improve recovery outcomes.

IMMUNE SUPPORT

Supporting the immune system is essential for maintaining overall health and protecting the body against infections and diseases. Natural remedies such as astragalus and reishi mushroom have been traditionally used to strengthen and enhance immune function. These remedies are known for their immune-boosting properties and ability to improve overall health.

ASTRAGALUS

Overview: Astragalus (Astragalus membranaceus) is a traditional Chinese herb known for its powerful immune-boosting properties. It has been used for centuries to enhance the body's natural defense mechanisms.

Key Benefits:

- **Strengthens the Immune System:** Astragalus boosts the immune system by increasing the production and activity of white blood cells, which are essential for fighting off infections.
- **Antiviral Properties:** Astragalus has antiviral properties that help protect against viral infections and reduce the severity and duration of colds and flu.
- **Anti-inflammatory Effects:** Astragalus reduces inflammation in the body, promoting overall health and supporting the immune system's ability to respond to threats.

Usage Recommendations:

- **Forms:** Astragalus is available in various forms, including capsules, tablets, tinctures, and teas.
- **Dosage:** For immune support, a common dosage is 250-500 mg of astragalus extract taken 2-3 times daily. It is advisable to consult a healthcare provider for the appropriate dosage based on individual health needs.

REISHI MUSHROOM

Overview: Reishi mushroom (Ganoderma lucidum) is a medicinal mushroom known for its immune-enhancing and overall health-promoting properties. It has been used in traditional Chinese medicine for thousands of years.

Key Benefits:

- **Enhances Immune Function:** Reishi mushroom boosts the immune system by increasing the activity of various immune cells, including macrophages, natural killer cells, and T-cells.

- **Supports Overall Health:** Reishi mushroom contains polysaccharides, triterpenes, and other compounds that promote overall health and longevity. It helps to reduce fatigue, improve sleep, and enhance mental clarity.

- **Anti-inflammatory and Antioxidant Properties:** Reishi mushroom has strong anti-inflammatory and antioxidant effects, which help to protect the body from chronic diseases and support overall immune health.

Usage Recommendations:

- **Forms:** Reishi mushroom is available in various forms, including capsules, tablets, extracts, and teas.
- **Dosage:** For immune support, a common dosage is 1,000-2,000 mg of reishi mushroom extract taken daily. It is advisable to consult a healthcare provider for the appropriate dosage and form.

Considerations:

- **Safety:** Both astragalus and reishi mushroom are

generally safe when used as directed. However, individuals with certain medical conditions or those taking specific medications should consult a healthcare provider before use. Astragalus may interact with immune-suppressing medications, and reishi mushroom should be used with caution by individuals with bleeding disorders or those taking blood-thinning medications.

- **Allergic Reactions:** Some people may experience allergic reactions or sensitivity to astragalus or reishi mushroom. It is important to monitor your body's response and consult a healthcare provider if any adverse effects occur.

Conclusion:

Astragalus and reishi mushroom are effective natural remedies for supporting immune health. Astragalus strengthens the immune system by boosting white blood cell production and activity, while reishi mushroom enhances immune function and overall health through its anti-inflammatory and antioxidant properties. Incorporating these natural remedies into your health routine, with appropriate dosages and professional guidance, can help maintain a strong immune system and improve overall well-being.

BRAIN HEALTH

Maintaining brain health is essential for cognitive function, memory, and overall mental well-being. Natural remedies such as ginkgo biloba and lion's mane mushroom have been traditionally used to enhance cognitive function and support brain health. These remedies are known for their ability to improve memory, promote nerve growth, and protect the brain.

GINKGO BILOBA

Overview: Ginkgo biloba is an ancient tree species whose leaves have been used in traditional medicine for thousands of years. It is renowned for its cognitive-enhancing properties.

Key Benefits:

- **Improves Cognitive Function:** Ginkgo biloba enhances cognitive performance, including memory, attention, and executive functions. It works by improving blood circulation to the brain and enhancing oxygen and nutrient delivery.
- **Enhances Memory:** Ginkgo biloba has been shown to improve both short-term and long-term memory, making it beneficial for individuals experiencing memory decline.
- **Neuroprotective Effects:** Ginkgo biloba contains potent antioxidants that protect brain cells from oxidative stress and damage, supporting overall brain health and reducing the risk of neurodegenerative diseases.

Usage Recommendations:

- **Forms:** Ginkgo biloba is available in various forms, including capsules, tablets, extracts, and teas.
- **Dosage:** For cognitive enhancement and memory improvement, a common dosage is 120-240 mg of ginkgo biloba extract taken daily, divided into two or three doses. It is advisable to consult a healthcare provider for the appropriate dosage based on individual health needs.

LION'S MANE MUSHROOM

Overview: Lion's mane mushroom (Hericium erinaceus) is a medicinal mushroom known for its unique appearance and cognitive health benefits. It has been used in traditional Chinese medicine for its neuroprotective and cognitive-enhancing properties.

Key Benefits:

- **Promotes Nerve Growth:** Lion's mane mushroom stimulates the production of nerve growth factor (NGF), a protein essential for the growth, maintenance, and survival of nerve cells. This supports brain health and cognitive function.
- **Enhances Cognitive Health:** Regular consumption of lion's mane mushroom can improve cognitive functions such as memory, focus, and mental clarity. It is particularly beneficial for preventing age-related cognitive decline.
- **Neuroprotective Properties:** Lion's mane mushroom protects the brain from oxidative stress and inflammation, which can help reduce the risk of neurodegenerative diseases such as Alzheimer's and Parkinson's.

Usage Recommendations:

- **Forms:** Lion's mane mushroom is available in various forms, including capsules, tablets, powders, and extracts.
- **Dosage:** For cognitive health and nerve growth, a common dosage is 500-1,000 mg of lion's mane mushroom extract

taken daily. It is best to consult a healthcare provider for specific dosage recommendations.

Considerations:

- **Safety:** Both ginkgo biloba and lion's mane mushroom are generally safe when used as directed. However, individuals with certain medical conditions or those taking specific medications should consult a healthcare provider before use. Ginkgo biloba may interact with blood-thinning medications and should be used with caution by individuals with bleeding disorders. Lion's mane mushroom should be used cautiously by individuals with allergies to mushrooms.
- **Side Effects:** Some people may experience side effects such as digestive upset, headache, or allergic reactions. It is important to monitor your body's response and consult a healthcare provider if any adverse effects occur.

Conclusion:

Ginkgo biloba and lion's mane mushroom are effective natural remedies for supporting brain health. Ginkgo biloba improves cognitive function and memory by enhancing blood circulation and providing neuroprotective effects. Lion's mane mushroom promotes nerve growth and cognitive health through its stimulation of nerve growth factor and neuroprotective properties. Incorporating these natural remedies into your health routine, with appropriate dosages and professional guidance, can help maintain cognitive function, improve memory, and support overall brain health.

HORMONAL SUPPORT

Maintaining hormonal balance is crucial for overall health and well-being, especially for women experiencing hormonal fluctuations during menopause or menstruation. Natural remedies such as black cohosh and evening primrose oil have been traditionally used to support hormonal health and alleviate related symptoms.

BLACK COHOSH

Overview: Black cohosh (Actaea racemosa) is a plant native to North America that has been used for centuries to treat various women's health issues, particularly those related to menopause.

Key Benefits:

- **Alleviates Menopausal Symptoms:** Black cohosh is particularly effective in reducing symptoms associated with menopause, such as hot flashes, night sweats, and mood swings. It works by mimicking the effects of estrogen in the body, helping to balance hormone levels.
- **Supports Hormonal Balance:** By acting on estrogen receptors, black cohosh helps to stabilize hormonal fluctuations, providing relief from menopausal discomforts.
- **Improves Sleep and Mood:** Black cohosh can help improve sleep quality and reduce anxiety and depression, which are common during menopause.

Usage Recommendations:

- **Forms:** Black cohosh is available in various forms, including capsules, tablets, tinctures, and teas.
- **Dosage:** For alleviating menopausal symptoms, a common dosage is 20-40 mg of black cohosh extract taken twice daily. It is advisable to consult a healthcare provider for the appropriate dosage based on individual health needs.

EVENING PRIMROSE OIL

Overview: Evening primrose oil (Oenothera biennis) is extracted from the seeds of the evening primrose plant. It is rich in gamma-linolenic acid (GLA), an omega-6 fatty acid that plays a key role in hormonal balance.

Key Benefits:

- **Balances Hormones:** Evening primrose oil helps to balance hormones by providing essential fatty acids that support the production and regulation of hormones. It is beneficial for women experiencing hormonal imbalances, particularly those related to PMS and menopause.
- **Reduces PMS Symptoms:** Evening primrose oil is effective in reducing symptoms of premenstrual syndrome (PMS), including breast tenderness, mood swings, bloating, and irritability.
- **Supports Skin Health:** The GLA in evening primrose oil helps to maintain healthy skin by reducing inflammation and improving skin moisture. It is particularly beneficial for individuals with hormonal acne.

Usage Recommendations:

- **Forms:** Evening primrose oil is available in various forms, including capsules, soft gels, and liquid oil.
- **Dosage:** For balancing hormones and reducing PMS symptoms, a common dosage is 500-1,000 mg of evening primrose oil taken twice daily. It is advisable to consult a

healthcare provider for the appropriate dosage and form.

Considerations:

- **Safety:** Both black cohosh and evening primrose oil are generally safe when used as directed. However, individuals with certain medical conditions or those taking specific medications should consult a healthcare provider before use. Black cohosh should be used with caution by individuals with liver conditions, and evening primrose oil should be used cautiously by those with epilepsy or bleeding disorders.
- **Side Effects:** Some people may experience side effects such as digestive upset, headache, or allergic reactions. It is important to monitor your body's response and consult a healthcare provider if any adverse effects occur.

Conclusion:

Black cohosh and evening primrose oil are effective natural remedies for supporting hormonal health. Black cohosh alleviates menopausal symptoms by balancing estrogen levels and reducing hot flashes, night sweats, and mood swings. Evening primrose oil balances hormones and reduces PMS symptoms by providing essential fatty acids that support hormone production and regulation. Incorporating these natural remedies into your health routine, with appropriate dosages and professional guidance, can help maintain hormonal balance and improve overall well-being.

GENERAL WELLNESS

Supporting general wellness is essential for maintaining overall health and preventing chronic diseases. Natural remedies such as holy basil and sea buckthorn are known for their broad-spectrum health benefits, including stress reduction, immune support, and antioxidant properties.

HOLY BASIL

Overview: Holy basil (Ocimum sanctum), also known as Tulsi, is an adaptogenic herb widely used in Ayurvedic medicine. It is renowned for its ability to reduce stress and support overall health.

Key Benefits:

- **Reduces Stress:** Holy basil helps the body adapt to stress by balancing cortisol levels and supporting adrenal function. It promotes relaxation and reduces anxiety, making it effective for managing stress-related conditions.
- **Supports Immune Health:** Holy basil has immunomodulatory properties that help to strengthen the immune system and improve resistance to infections.
- **Anti-inflammatory and Antioxidant Properties:** Holy basil contains compounds such as eugenol and rosmarinic acid, which have anti-inflammatory and antioxidant effects. These properties help protect the body from oxidative stress and inflammation, promoting overall health.

Usage Recommendations:

- **Forms:** Holy basil is available in various forms, including capsules, tablets, teas, and tinctures.
- **Dosage:** For general wellness and stress reduction, a common dosage is 300-600 mg of holy basil extract taken once or twice daily. Drinking holy basil tea 1-2 times daily is also beneficial. It is advisable to consult a healthcare provider for the appropriate dosage and form.

SEA BUCKTHORN

Overview: Sea buckthorn (Hippophae rhamnoides) is a nutrient-dense plant known for its high content of vitamins, minerals, and antioxidants. It is particularly valued for its ability to support overall health and wellness.

Key Benefits:

- **Rich in Vitamins and Antioxidants:** Sea buckthorn is a rich source of vitamins A, C, E, and several B vitamins. It also contains flavonoids, carotenoids, and omega fatty acids, which provide strong antioxidant protection against free radicals.
- **Supports Skin Health:** The high vitamin C and E content in sea buckthorn helps to promote healthy skin by supporting collagen production and protecting against UV-induced damage. It is often used to improve skin hydration and reduce signs of aging.
- **Enhances Immune Function:** Sea buckthorn boosts the immune system by providing essential nutrients that support immune cell function and reduce inflammation.
- **Promotes Heart Health:** The omega-7 fatty acids in sea buckthorn support cardiovascular health by reducing cholesterol levels and improving blood vessel function.

Usage Recommendations:

- **Forms:** Sea buckthorn is available in various forms, including oils, capsules, juices, and powders.
- **Dosage:** For overall health, a common recommendation is to take 500-1,000 mg of sea buckthorn oil daily or 1-2 tablespoons of sea buckthorn juice. It is advisable

to consult a healthcare provider for specific dosage recommendations.

Considerations:

- **Safety:** Both holy basil and sea buckthorn are generally safe when used as directed. However, individuals with certain medical conditions or those taking specific medications should consult a healthcare provider before use. Holy basil may interact with blood-thinning medications, and sea buckthorn should be used with caution by individuals with low blood pressure or bleeding disorders.

- **Side Effects:** Some people may experience side effects such as digestive upset or allergic reactions. It is important to monitor your body's response and consult a healthcare provider if any adverse effects occur.

Conclusion:

Holy basil and sea buckthorn are effective natural remedies for supporting general wellness. Holy basil reduces stress and supports overall health through its adaptogenic and antioxidant properties. Sea buckthorn, rich in vitamins and antioxidants, enhances immune function, promotes skin health, and supports cardiovascular health. Incorporating these natural remedies into your wellness routine, with appropriate dosages and professional guidance, can help maintain overall health and improve quality of life.

ANTIMICROBIAL PROPERTIES

Natural remedies such as oregano oil and thyme have been traditionally used for their powerful antimicrobial properties. These remedies are effective against various bacterial and fungal infections, supporting overall health and well-being by helping to prevent and treat infections.

OREGANO OIL

Overview: Oregano oil (Origanum vulgare) is a potent essential oil known for its strong antimicrobial properties. It is effective against a wide range of bacterial and fungal infections.

Key Benefits:

- **Antibacterial Properties:** Oregano oil contains compounds such as carvacrol and thymol, which have been shown to inhibit the growth of various bacteria, including E. coli, Staphylococcus aureus, and Pseudomonas aeruginosa.

- **Antifungal Properties:** Oregano oil is effective against fungal infections, including Candida albicans, which causes yeast infections. Its antifungal properties help to inhibit the growth and spread of fungi.

- **Supports Immune Health:** Oregano oil boosts the immune system by enhancing the body's ability to fight off infections. It can be used both topically and internally to support immune function and prevent infections.

Usage Recommendations:

- **Forms:** Oregano oil is available in various forms, including essential oil, capsules, and liquid extracts.

- **Dosage:** For internal use, a common dosage is 2-4 drops of oregano oil diluted in water or juice, taken up to three times daily. For topical use, dilute oregano oil with a carrier oil (such as coconut or olive oil) before applying it to the affected area. It is advisable to consult a healthcare provider for specific dosage recommendations and to ensure safe use.

THYME

Overview: Thyme (Thymus vulgaris) is a herb known for its strong antimicrobial properties. It has been used traditionally to treat various infections due to its ability to combat bacteria, fungi, and viruses.

Key Benefits:

- **Antimicrobial Properties:** Thyme contains thymol and carvacrol, which have potent antimicrobial effects. These compounds help to inhibit the growth of bacteria, fungi, and viruses, making thyme effective in treating a variety of infections.

- **Supports Respiratory Health:** Thyme is often used to treat respiratory infections such as bronchitis and sore throats due to its antimicrobial and anti-inflammatory properties. It helps to clear mucus and reduce inflammation in the respiratory tract.

- **Boosts Immune Function:** Thyme supports the immune system by enhancing the body's natural defense mechanisms, helping to prevent and fight infections.

Usage Recommendations:

- **Forms:** Thyme is available in various forms, including fresh or dried herb, essential oil, capsules, and tinctures.

- **Dosage:** For treating infections, a common recommendation is to drink thyme tea made from 1-2 teaspoons of dried thyme leaves steeped in hot water, up to three times daily. For topical use, dilute thyme essential oil with a carrier oil before applying it to the affected area. It is advisable to consult a healthcare provider for specific dosage recommendations.

Considerations:

- **Safety:** Both oregano oil and thyme are generally safe when used as directed. However, individuals with certain medical conditions or those taking specific medications should consult a healthcare provider before use. Oregano oil should be used with caution by individuals with allergies to plants in the Lamiaceae family and should be properly diluted to avoid skin irritation. Thyme should be used with caution by individuals with hormone-sensitive conditions or those taking blood-thinning medications.
- **Side Effects:** Some people may experience side effects such as digestive upset, skin irritation, or allergic reactions. It is important to monitor your body's response and consult a healthcare provider if any adverse effects occur.

Conclusion:

Oregano oil and thyme are effective natural remedies for their antimicrobial properties. Oregano oil is potent against various bacterial and fungal infections and supports immune health. Thyme, with its strong antimicrobial properties, is effective in treating infections and supporting respiratory health. Incorporating these natural remedies into your health routine, with appropriate dosages and professional guidance, can help prevent and treat infections, promoting overall health and well-being.

SUMMARY

In exploring the vast world of natural remedies, this book has been a journey through time-honored traditions and modern discoveries, all aimed at enhancing our health and well-being through nature's bounty. From the soothing effects of chamomile tea to the potent anti-inflammatory properties of turmeric, each chapter dives into the unique benefits of herbs, roots, and other natural ingredients that our ancestors have trusted for centuries.

We've covered a range of topics essential to everyday wellness: boosting the immune system with elderberry and echinacea, supporting digestive health with ginger and peppermint, and managing pain with the likes of turmeric and willow bark. Each remedy is presented with its key benefits, practical usage recommendations, and important considerations to keep in mind.

For those dealing with respiratory issues, we've looked at the power of mullein and oregano oil, while cardiovascular health is supported by the incredible properties of garlic and hawthorn. When it comes to energy and vitality, ginseng and maca root have stood out, while resveratrol and ashwagandha offer promising benefits for anti-aging and longevity.

Navigating allergies has been made easier with stinging nettle and quercetin, while headaches and migraines find relief in feverfew and peppermint oil. Joint and muscle pain can be managed with the help of arnica and capsaicin, and liver health is supported by milk thistle and dandelion root. We've even delved into the importance of kidney health with cranberry and nettle.

The book doesn't shy away from mental health either, exploring how lavender and chamomile can ease anxiety and promote sleep. For those looking to support their sexual health, maca root and tribulus terrestris provide natural solutions. Hair health can be improved with rosemary and horsetail, while bone and joint health benefit from boswellia and hyaluronic acid.

Detoxification is simplified with burdock root and chlorella, and for urinary health, D-mannose and corn silk offer effective remedies. When it comes to wound healing, honey and gotu kola are standout solutions, and for brain health, ginkgo biloba and lion's mane mushroom show incredible promise.

In terms of hormonal balance, black cohosh and evening primrose oil are discussed for their roles in alleviating menopausal symptoms and balancing hormones. General wellness is rounded out with holy basil and sea buckthorn, providing stress reduction and nutritional support.

Finally, the book explores the antimicrobial properties of oregano oil and thyme, offering natural ways to combat infections.

Throughout this book, the goal has been to provide you with practical, reliable, and natural ways to improve your health. It's been a personal journey for me to gather and share this knowledge, hoping it can make a difference in your life as it has in mine. Embracing the power of nature can lead to a healthier, more balanced life, and I'm excited for you to experience these benefits firsthan